GRIGORI GRABOVOI

Selected Lectures

Jelezky publishing, Hamburg 2011

Jelezky publishing, Hamburg
www.jelezky-media.com

English 1st Edition, july 2011
(1st Edition)

English Translation: Lingua Communications Translation Services, USA

Further information about the contents:
SVET centre, Hamburg

www.svet-centre.eu, info@svet-centre.eu

ISBN: 978-3-943110-11-1

Medical Disclaimer

The information within this book is intended as reference material only, and not as medical or professional advice. Information contained herein is intended to give you the tools to make informed decisions about your lifestyle and health. It should not be used as a substitute for any treatment that has been prescribed or recommended by your qualified doctor. Do not stop taking any medication unless advised by your qualified doctor to do otherwise. The author and publisher are not healthcare professionals, and expressly disclaim any responsibility for any adverse effects occurring as a result of the use of suggestions or information herein. This book is offered as current information available about health management, for your own education and enjoyment.

As always, never begin a health program without first consulting a qualified healthcare professional.

Your use of this book indicates your agreement to these terms.

Thank You!

Contents

Individual Lecture Courses

Moscow, 1999-2000

Lecture 1

In this lecture I set forth at the beginning the principles of specialization, based on the fact that every individual has his own status of information at the level of common connections; specifically every person has access to the control structure, practically, which is connected to all the processes in the World. So it happens that an individual as a component of the World participates in the control either voluntarily, consciously or, for example, just due to the fact of his existence. So, by the fact of his existence, by the level of creating the individual, which includes physical matter, the human Soul, Spirit, consciousness, mind — that is, all the categories pertaining to the personality, the individual may at a certain level apply maximum effort so as to realize his potential in my system of salvation.

Since now the matter in question is the possibility of global destruction, the system of salvation is in fact the most adequate reaction of the individual. Therefore, what I am saying with respect to specialization is that I am announcing the structure of personality, the system of your information, through which you can exert maximum control. And you do that periodically, for example, as a result of some situations, for example, through direct conscious control, or in your sleep, or sometimes without thinking. Nevertheless, what I am saying is aimed at those things that must be saved, in the technologies of salvation, in any circumstances. In other words, one must know how to save it, even if there is no prior experience. This technology is based precisely on this practice.

And in this regard, what I am saying, for you it turns out that you must see ahead the event already optimized, that is, ahead you must already see the situation where for you everything is normalized. And this vision ahead in fact determines your specialization, which is: you control information through the structure of discreet access to intermediary areas of information. In other words, for example, there is information of current time exists: in an hour, in a second, in a millisecond — this may be information of future time, but in the same way as for the time past. But that's how you, when you exert control in accordance with your specialization, you control to the maximum when, for example, you record the information of current time; let us assume it is now 9:58 pm, and the next information you view as the connection between information of the current time and information of the future via the path of some events, for example, the second hand has moved — something happened in the external environment and the internal.

So, your control involves the fact that you have access to every event continuously from one point, which you select arbitrarily. This can be presented in the following way: since the event of current time and future time are connected by a certain, let's say, sequence, sort of a thread, or in the form of links of a chain, and you can have access to any structure of the chain, both sequentially to each element or to all of them simultaneously. So that is the level of your specialization. At that level, you can control the macrosystem to the maximum extent. As I explained, you are part of the World; therefore, control at the macrolevel is performed with maximum speed in places where you know the principles of your, practically, functioning at the transition, where your information transitions into the information of control of all the connections of the World. And this transition of yours, it lies in the fact that you, using consciousness, enter into the area of discrete control.

In order to apply this knowledge to oneself, it is possible to look at a specific situation: if, for example, some unfavorable event occurs to a person whom you know; then, in order to optimize the event, that is, dispel the possible negative impact occurring due to that event; or there are situations when the entire event needs to be changed radically, that is, to make it so that it, for example, is not there, did not happen, or had a less pronounced effect in the past. But when we are talking about, first and foremost, making the consequences of the event, let's say, optimized and not so negative as they could have been without interference, the matter in question is that this system of access, it implies: first (1st principle) — this is after all maximum status optimization. So it means that you must regulate the event to the extent to which it is possible —optimize to the maximum extent, that is, there should not be any intermediary links here.

Comment of an attendee: So, I should be seeing a video clip of the optimal result.

Grigori Petrovich.: Seeing is one thing. And the second thing, this is the kind of ideology you must have: suppose that a patient comes with stage 4 cancer; the impulse to the patient must be made that we are talking about complete healing, and not improvements. If we are looking at very serious, life-threatening injuries, restoration is still the objective. If we are talking about an event where, for example, we see a situation, let's say, a specific one, where a person was run over, it means that we need to the maximum extent improve the condition of all the parties: first, it is possible to unlock this factor in the past, and also to reduce the structure of the conflict level; second, as the facts are already in place and the status of the event is reinforced, then the consequences should be minimized through the system of discrete access, as I explained.

That is, for example, to break down the whole event into a chain, from which they will start branching off, like in a hierarchy, into the possible combinations that would follow; and through the system of either instant access to all events, that is, sending an internal impulse to all the events at once, or to a specific event; and alternating them in this manner: to all and then to a specific one, to all, etc. — alternate them internally. This way, you minimize and optimize it, that is, balance it in line with the overall harmony, where in principle people do not suffer, for example. And taking into account that there really are some situations when people are not to blame, so then what you have to do is simply harmonize it. To do this, you will be using this impulse system. It is similar to what you see with, say, flashes of light: a ray may hit one link, or a flash may illuminate all the links. It is the same thing here. That is what it should be like, the flashes of your consciousness. Since you are already in the control sphere, and as it works for you, you will see not possible theoretical developments, but the specific path of development, which, if you do not interfere, will proceed to develop that way. So when you do interfere, you will change it for the better. So that will be the training for a specific situation.

In continuation of this lecture, I would like to say that working with the material should continue by breaking it up into two components. The information presented on the audiotape should, in the course of this breakdown, be perceived from the center of this division. Or one can imagine it in the shape of a sphere, the information from this part of the lecture, and then take the same from the non-verbal level. Then, everything that you have collected, transfer to the level of factual information, that is, what corresponds to the World. That is, this factual level is, in practice, that very action where information is located corresponding to this part of the lecture, let's say, in the true structure of the World, and not at the level of thinking. Thinking is also a structure of the World; so the truth here is what brings us towards the specific action, in other words, towards the result.

Based on that, I will now tell you what is the axiomatic structure of the system of interconnections, aimed at the following: the requirements that your mind, your body, your personality set for yourself in order to have them adequately expressed in the society and in the overall system of the World. In this plane there are axioms, which are as follows:

Axiom one: If consciousness is part of the Soul, then the Soul can be reproduced by consciousness. And when we look at this axiom, there is immediately a second one, as a corollary to it; axiom two: Spiritual development is reproduction of the Soul via the consciousness of action. Through conscious action negative events can be transformed into normalized physical ones — it is as if you have corrected them in terms of information.

When we are talking about how to transform a thought, for example, into control, the way it works is that the thought, as a derivative of the body and Soul, (and we look at the body as a part of the Soul), transitions into control at the point where the Soul touches consciousness. So, the contact of the Soul with the consciousness is the point of reflection from the consciousness. When you become familiar with this terminology, having listened to it several times, you will see that consciousness is an infinite area, an infinite value, which is characterized by the fact that awareness of consciousness is a process of constructive and harmonious development. And when you, for example, take this development and apply it to the specialization under your system of redemption, then in there you see that development is the status that exists for you. That is, in principle it is realistic, if you look at yourself from the outside, that you are constantly in one and the same state. Therefore, development is the understanding of status, and the understanding of status is an element of consciousness. This completes my first lecture.

Lecture 2

The second lecture defines the laws of connection between the elements of consciousness and the elements of the Soul. In order to develop and apply the controlling clairvoyance in accordance with the technology of salvation, the elements of consciousness must be connected to the elements of the Soul on the basis of the special technology of transformation of the Soul, the structure of the Soul into the structure of consciousness. That is, the process initially comes from the level of the Soul, which is in fact the level of the Creator. So transformation of the structure of the Soul into the consciousness is a special technology which is reflected on a spiritual basis, but it is reflected in the form of action, which the spiritual basis exerts onto the consciousness. So I perform a special detailed breakdown and divide some... let's call them concepts of the World, so as to discover the essence, your controlling essence, but to discover it in such a way that you would already have the controlling clairvoyance, possess it, have the skills, for example, for healing if needed, or any irrational techniques from just having heard this material.

That is, now that you are listening to this material, the information is shaped around you in such a way; there is a so-called mantra principle and, based on this mantra principle, you in fact do it, that is, you in fact organize events. That is, when knowledge is transferred from the teacher to the student, not all the knowledge is transferred as words, but some words are given the status of control.

So, what I told you this time, in the first lecture and in the part of the lecture which we are going through now — this is the creation of a special level of information around you, which will create the optimal environment for you.

So, when we are talking about infinite time, which is seen, or you become aware of it via consciousness, you must understand: there is one simple fact, axiomatically, that in any case all the events of reality with people, or with some situations, need to be resolved — through the level of creation, since time is infinite, matter is infinite, space is infinite. It is still necessary to negotiate (similar to the way the ritual in the tea house is going on in Uzbekistan), on the basis of information or in real events, and not to use any rough methods of influence — physical or violent.

So, the principle is that once you know that, it immediately becomes obvious what to do. Suppose even if external circumstances are pushing one towards use of some methods which are perhaps more rough, one must know how to get out of this situation from the information standpoint. So this is a concept like… there is a concept of a miracle, some informational drastic growth, when internally you sort of offer all your problems upwards and receive the solution; that is, you are not destroying anyone, you are not touching anyone, but you receive the solution. On the information plane, yes, you can move something there, but on the other hand physically you have not touched anyone, or gone on to the next step, or if your preceding actions were there and they were negative, you sort of settled them on the information plane.

Then you can develop, and your personality can become infinite. That is, here, in the infinite development — that is what I present — complete restoration of the matter, then there you will see where the status of complete restoration of the matter is located. The thing is that what was necessary at the level of creating the necessary spiritual construct, I provided in this verbal status. The task is: at the initial stages to listen to this second lecture, without going into the detailed structure of the verbal component. That is, mostly what you need is to have a formed Spirit. Later the technology will be understandable even when presented in the form of words.

Lecture 3

This lecture is aimed at redefining information on the future, based on fragments which could be classified as information of the past. In order to perform these actions, it is necessary to single out the level of stability of the inherent form of information; that is, practically, to find a basis on which you have stability in terms of access. If you view the information in its infinite form, then any point is stable. But in order to define information in terms of targeted actions: you need to save someone from terrorists, you need to save a specific person, you need to cure someone from a disease, you need to generally resolve a personal or social problem, or any problem — then the point of stability is, in a geometric sense, the informational center of this problem. That is, as soon as you have formed the principle of stability from that position, the second principle of stability is to not be located, informationally, in its own substance, in that center, that is, to be located outside of the boundaries of that information. Having set those two points, the third principle will be that, having become aware of those two postulates, you are at the level of organizing the information of this event. Once you have arrived at the level of organizing the information, the action is forming the event base on the principle I have stated for forming the event by using the fragments of the past.

So, for this it is necessary to consider how a future event is formed. If we look at the entire body of information or, to put it simply, all the information, we shall see when we look at this information in depth and in detail, that information from the past flows into the information of the future. Here is the simplest example: a second ago, a building was standing; a second later, this building is, again, standing, so the way it works is that information, in principle, is sort of transferred. If we view the entire World as an infinite straight line, then the movement of time is similar to a plane which, at all times, crosses that line (we can say either a plane, or a three-dimensional space), and this moves at all times. Then it comes to the fact that in the interval of movement we can single out some microzone in which all this happens. Since all this is happening — there exist connections between the past and the future. So when you are building a future event, even if it is a hundred years ahead or even an infinity ahead, you can connect that event with that moving boundary, and so it will mean that you have transferred it into the structure of the past.

When you perform a transfer from the future to the past, a special technology exists there: first of all, the simplest way is to perform the transfer at the background level, that is, in the level of one's creation, when you are balanced, that is, you harmoniously exist everywhere. That is, you do not have an overconcentration with respect to this task, or a second, or a third one — you are harmonious everywhere and exist everywhere. Then the way it works is that the transition into the past is performed through your pituitary gland via a natural way of functioning of your consciousness. Because the pituitary gland is sort of the material representation of this boundary in the function of control over future events. The pituitary gland, the one in the brain I mean, is a specific physical formation, physical tissue. Therefore, when there is some future event in existence, when future events are perceived, and they are of the kind that you don't like and you want to change them, for some reason a signal is generated that is transmitted seemingly to the heart, or to the liver, or to the spleen. As they say: „I have a gut feeling, a fit of spleen", — these are the colloquial expressions. And it is related to the fact that some of the organs serve as the grouping centers in that boundary. And there is a very clear relation as to which organ can perceive an element of a future event how many years in advance.

This way, in order to see all the events ahead and form them, it is necessary simply to standardize the system of access to the organs which have that information for you, regarding the future, for example. So, the essence of this standardization of access is, again, the skill of transforming information from the past into a future fragment. Now I already create a global construct, so it is placed in space. So, in that space, for example, it is a multi-dimensional space, I bring up an understandable view: for example, a plane is flying. In the plane there is a seat and there is a pilot; and when the plane starts falling and weightlessness sets in, or turbulence, for example, then a third state will occur there, which is not in line with the flight objectives. So, the third state, which is not in line with the flight objectives — this is the state that requires more detailed control, for example, than the intended states. And so when you arrive at the state of control, for example, it must not be allowed for the plane to fall (it is similar to an off-nominal situation or potential catastrophe), then in that state, during diagnostics of that plane you will clearly see within it the sphere, which I partially described, that is, the sphere of the event. And the reason I said that one should not transfer the essence of one's consciousness, that is, you can see it with your perception, but do not transfer the essence of your consciousness inside. The essence of your consciousness is something that belongs to you, that relates to you.

Comment of an attendee: That is, one should not associate oneself with this event.

Grigori Petrovich: Do not transfer the essence into the center, but rather set another point outside...

Comment of an attendee: As if I am watching television.

Grigori Petrovich: Yes, from the outside, in another point which is somewhere outside: in the same plane or infinitely remote. And as soon as you set it — the plane will start leveling out, the circuit boards that have burnt out will reappear, etc. That is, this is the level of the balance, coming from the center of the event and level of your consciousness; this construct, in fact, is that very element of the World, which determines the structure of the past in the future.

This way, in order to single out the structure of the past in the future, knowing this construct, for example, you know the shapes, that a square has a certain design, a sphere has a certain design, so, you know the shape; when there is a large mass — land, forest, some kind of scaffolding is being built, there is construction work underway — then you can single out from there a fragment of a square, a fragment of a sphere, a circle, etc. It is the same thing here: when you know the design of the structure of the past-future; when you look into the future, you will always find there elements of the past, even if by simple perception. And the technique that I am teaching you, the point of it is that as soon as in the future you start looking for elements of the past, among other ways in a natural, harmonious way (to call it "automatically" would not be properly describing its content. Rather it is "harmoniously"). You become what you perceive at the level of your consciousness and controlling reality. That is, the very search of the past in the elements of the future already provides the harmonization that I talked about.

That is, there are quite specific technologies for the background level of control, when you, without overconcentration, in a natural, normal state, in the state of eternal functioning, in the state of eternal life, are capable of controlling any situation. In this case you are solving the true task of the Creator — creation of endless, eternal, indestructible life. That is, then you are moving in accordance with your design.

And now I am transitioning to the structure of spiritual control, where these principles lie in the basis of each action; that is, what is said with respect to technology and was to a significant extent aimed at awareness of consciousness, in this case on the spiritual basis — this is a minor element. The following comparison may be provided: there are computers (of course, it is a very schematic and approximate comparison, but nonetheless); if we take a floppy disk, then all the information from the floppy disk, that is, all the technology that is within that floppy disk, we can record onto a CD-ROM, where there can already be millions of such technologies.. So this CD-ROM — is the level of the spiritual, in this comparison.

To put it more simply, at the spiritual level information is so concentrated, that what I read now within this lecture in the way of technology for orienting one's consciousness and control via the consciousness at that point transitions to the level of already being in existence. That is, when you transition to the spiritual system, you meet the same things as already exist. And that is where the difference lies: when you perform here, you act: that is, for you it is still the result of action, in other words, it belongs to the future. At the spiritual level you always encounter the already existent; that is, the Spirit exists everywhere — both in the past and in the future. So, in order to understand your spiritual foundation and transition to the Soul — that which creates everything where you are created, where you exist always and forever. That is, in fact, to find yourself there means that you are indestructible.

So it means that here one needs to proceed from a completely different standpoint, from a completely different principle of perception and a different principle of physical sense of self and self-consciousness. That is, here you should be guided by the fact that in reality you are actually selecting just an element with which you have been familiar for a long time. So hence the working technology on the basis of the beginning of spiritual forming, where the Spirit is formed. It is not the same as spiritual formation: you are studying something, developing — this is different; specifically, where your Spirit is forming on the basis of information. There you work as if at a level with which you are very familiar. That is, there is that spiritual feeling of kinship, spiritual closeness, spiritual understanding — there is such a concept. For example, this picture is understandable for your Soul, you realize spiritually. Why? First, it may be because you are, within the structure of organization, spiritual in nature, and that makes it clear for you.

As soon as you come farther, where the Spirit connects to the mental aspects — with the mind, with consciousness — so it means that you are already moving, advancing into the structure of connections. Then you start analyzing. How is logic created? You could see that absolutely clearly, if you want to. Where does the logical phase pass and why it is connected to the Soul in one way, and in a different way with the spiritual level? What, within the structure of connections, is the mind and what is the sign of the presence of the mind? That is, you can find all these answers. In this case it is not the objective. The objective is that you should correctly and in principle rightly find in the spiritual sphere the same thing that you find in the sphere of consciousness. Then, crossing over that, you come to the Soul, to that on the basis of which everything that is yours is created. That is, the Creator created the Soul, and that is what the physical body is - a part of the Soul. Therefore, you can, knowing the connections between the consciousness and the Spirit, see the principles on which it is built, and that means to reach oneself, always recreate oneself through consciousness, that is, through one's desire. And since it is so, you can naturally control in a constructive form any process which can be in a remote point from you, either in the past or in the future. Therefore, on a spiritual basis the past contained in the future is a segment which relates to the point of connection of your consciousness: you are your Spirit.

Once you have listened to this lecture, you will be at this point in reality. In the future, your task is: to locate it in the level where you want to exert control. Even just locating this point at the right level already provides control. And therefore this is again the same very level where you - at the background level, at the level of your organization, at the level of harmony - can exert control, that is, in general, without performing any visible actions. You know this point; you take it, locate it, and that's where the control already begins.

Lecture 4

This lecture defines control of the area of the Spirit or, in other words, of the spiritual area via the status of the Soul. In this case, the status of the Soul means that the principle of the Soul is eternity. That is, since the Soul is eternal, it turns out how one can change the structure of the Soul from the standpoint of the concept of dynamics so as to control the spiritual area further: connect it with the consciousness, with an event, etc.

So, using the status of the Soul, control is done through the structure; first and foremost, this is changing impulse forms. I will introduce this concept. Impulse form — this is something that exists as an impulse and has a specific form or shape, but at the same time, when the impulse form appears, it does not compromise the static form of the main object. There is a law of the Universe which says that the originally existing status will always be preserved.

This law can be traced in many principles of reality, for example: a second has passed; everything that remained in the past, in principle, is considered unreachable, etc. That is an example of what kind of laws there are. This is development of the principle of eternity on the structure of dynamics. So now I transfer this principle so that you have a precise methodology of control through immobility of the static state of the Soul.

It turns out, in order to effect the transfer, this impulse needs to be generated, but in doing so one must use the existing reality. And the example which I provided, that it is believed that it is impossible to enter the past using the physical method, for example, says that there exists a spiritual method. And when we transfer some informational object into future events, we always use the transition of the informational or spiritual plane. That is, actually, when it is a question of the status of the Soul, one can say that in this status everything exists simultaneously.

And when you transition already to control of the existing, it turns out a control task arises of a completely different order. It is approximately the same as, say, the following task if you transfer it to the plane of perception of physical objects: there is a table and table surface. How can you control the surface of the table within the framework of its existence? That is, how is control possible? It is clear that if, from the standpoint of physical reality, you need to connect one element of the table to another, it is necessary, let us assume, to connect pieces of the table using instruments; but in order to connect them in your imagination, in principle, you don't need to do anything. You can just imagine them connected. When you establish the connection in the imagination, that is, in thought, and transfer it to some object, for example, a physical object, like the edge of the table, you could saw it a little and move the particles onto the other side; that means it works for you, that at first you thought it through, that is, in fact you created an image somewhere. And now there is a more detailed design: where is this image created? If it is in the status in which you are working at the level of the Soul, everything exists at all times in all interconnections. Therefore, you are working at the level of action. That is, I in this case designate action, work, as a separate status attribute of reality through which you can exert control, knowing that it exists. That is, if for this table, for example, we set the element of action to the side, then we are not sawing anything, but we can think — this is an action as well. Thus, in action there exists a level of control of some status, for example, the physical one, and the level of action, even without action in another plane, in the plane of understanding it. For example, we may not be sawing a piece off, but we may be aware of it in thought.

Further, when we pass to the level of the Soul, it turns out that this principle

„action without action“ actually exists at the basis of organizing the consequence of control of the Soul, specifically the outcome of control of the Soul. Because, in order to come to the original attribute, it is necessary to know how the Creator created, that is, the technology of creation by the Creator. So, this is the level of the consciousness about which I am talking now, and it determines actually the connection of the Soul with its own elements, to put it simply. It is even possible to say not „simply“, but in a more technical way, because in principle there is no concept of simplicity there, but the concept of word and action. So, in order to use the discovered principle for controlling the spiritual basis, it is important to understand that this transmitting structure between the elements of the Soul - that it is a spiritual basis. That is, in this definition the Spirit is an element of the dynamics of the Soul. It is the same as if you perform a physical action and the wind rises, or perform an action using the physical level, then the Spirit is an element of the dynamics of the Soul.

That is, at this level of understanding, but not in the plane of movement per se, but in the plane of the outline of the Soul in a predefined area, we are coming to an understanding of consciousness. That is, in what way do you perceive with consciousness, in the state of logical contemplation to perceive reality, so as to realize this status of the Soul? That is, when you work putting your Soul into it, that is, using the Soul, then this work is harmonized throughout the entirety of time-space, that is, it will be harmonious in any case. And so it goes that you need to transfer the level of the element of consciousness to the status of the work of the Soul. So this transition already has the same structure, as in information of the Spirit, that is, within the spiritual foundation elements are contained that are outcomes of consciousness.

I am showing a rather unusual perspective here. The thing is, I am showing not how sufficiently clearly the Spirit can modify the consciousness depending on the condition of the Spirit, and the perception of the conscious changes —

that is clear to everybody. But here I am showing a different element: that the spiritual structure contains within it an element that comes from consciousness. That is, if you think this way, simply contemplate from the consciousness to Spirit, then we shall again come to an area of consciousness, but this time it is already one which comes directly in contact with the area of the Soul. That is, actually this method is standardized, and it states that everything is in contact with the Soul: consciousness, body, Spirit, physical reality, etc.

Thus, by announcing the essence of the Soul as the basis of the Universe, which it is, because it is created by the Creator, it is possible to transition to the way in which any element, in the standardized understanding thereof, is controlled by the Soul. There is a saying, for example: „a developed Soul". Why is it developed? Thus, the principle development of the Soul can come from the Creator, but the principle of development may also come from the degree of development, for example, of the consciousness, which is also set forth by the Creator. That is, when the development from Creator is in progress and the things that He had put in the thought of that creature, then the divine principle of eternity ensues. So again, it is not even a recurrence, but again announcing eternity as an element of every movement.

Thus, I have derived in this case the following verbal formula: when eternity is an element of movement, we arrive at the status of the Creator. That is, the control task is to attain the understanding with what the Creator entrusted an individual personality in each period, for example, with respect to consciousness, to the Soul. An individual personality is a complex concept, containing the Soul, body, consciousness, etc. So, in this case, when we are following the development of the World, we must understand better the status set by the Creator. So, knowledge that comes from the Creator is the direct knowledge you have. And knowledge that comes from the Creator is what you have, including in physical reality: the fact that you are moving, you have certain plans, you implement them. This is happening — so that comes from the Creator as well. That is, actually by connecting the profound true knowledge that comes from the Creator with respect to the eternity of development with what you have in reality, that confirms the fact of your actions that come from the Creator; thus we have an intermediary level, which tells us what knowledge we can have that will be given as the next step, based on what we have now. That means that in fact I have established a law which exists at the level of understanding.

So I am proceeding to the next area — the laws of understanding which exist and their development. That is, any development may be correct, knowing that the environment is oriented in such a way as to develop all your actions in accordance with the status of the Creator. And the Creator obviously has set this status unequivocally, and to a large extent He has already set it with elements of teaching this status. It is simple then — you just need to know where those elements are contained. And when we are talking about a developed Soul — this means it is developed in the area of knowledge, that is, in the area of interaction, as a rule. That is, for example, they say: the Soul is developed, he is soulfully developed, he has a developed Soul, because he interacts in the right way. That means he understands the structure of action, the structure of contact with another environment. And therefore, the broader the development of the Soul is, for example, for Jesus Christ it was developed to encompass all people, the entire World, and therefore, He is part of them as well.

The consequence from that is that the path of movement towards the Creator — this is the path to eternity. And the meaning of this movement is: it then unites the status of the consciousness and status of the Spirit. That is, where there is eternity, elements transform according to a standardized principle; that is, an element of the Spirit becomes an element of consciousness. There is unification of completely different perspectives in understanding, because the word in the course of its infinite development becomes the word of truth of the Creator. For example, in ancient Tibet, it was believed that by saying this word, he, for example, a lama, contacts God directly. But it was a very long word sometimes. That is, it shows that transition of the word forms is of fundamental importance. So, when you are listening to this lecture, the transition via the sound "o", information before the sound "o" and after the sound "o" is the transition into a niche where the word phase merges with action. That is, word and action — that will be one. And so when „In the beginning was the Word..." — the action was also the word. That is, from this viewpoint, the word „eternity" defines the action, the real existence of eternity.

That is, in order to find the mechanism of controlling events and apply it instantaneously, it is necessary to have the status, developed in such a way that you always predetermine events towards the positive side. In fact, I have now brought you towards that status level, and I have done so by activating among other methods the technology of working through words, when, being there, you have definitely been saved, and saved others. That is, there is that system of action embedded in the training; it presumes the same form of dissemination to others, to the self in the future, etc. That is, salvation does not mean a probable possibility; it means only an unequivocal and real structure which is implementable because, among other reasons, it has already been implemented.

Here I will again resort to technology and show why it is completed: because in the future you will have implemented it. And so the alignment of the future with the present provides the spiritual status. As it turns out, when we take an element of the future and align it with the present, the result is an element of the Spirit. So, when the Spirit is created as an element of an event, then you can see that the event is present in your own Spirit. And in this case control is rather simple: it is sufficient to just change the spiritual content, which comes from your own Soul. Only those solutions which you have had for a long time, they are contained in an element of the future. But as for the element of the future, if we regard the World not only as coming from you, but when we look how, on the fundamental principle of common interrelations, for example, your Spirit is formed from the space-time standpoint. So, from the space-time standpoint, the element of the Spirit is formed when the future is combined with the present. If you take the future with the past, you will receive the element of consciousness. So then the present will be designated as the reaction — this is the element of consciousness.

That is, in these phrases it is possible to find very simple reactive technologies, but according to the control status of salvation that has already been accomplished. That is, in this case, when you know that, it means that you are already invulnerable, that is, you come to the structure of your own organization. And when the structure of your own organization starts growing further, you understand further that, for example, if you take an element of your future, then your future exists in the informational plane in the same way as an element of your Spirit. So, when you take your past, the element of the Spirit already existed there, and you were there. In order to become eternal and not deteriorate, all you need is in this element to simply copy your existence, for example, from whatever age you need onto the element of the future, that is, restructure your spiritual basis in this way. So in that status you are already there. But since the Spirit exists in the future and what it has there is not just that it is there, but there also exists the reverse mechanism: from the connection in thought, that is, a mental connection of the future with the past, you can receive consciousness; but from the connection of the future with the current, you will receive the Spirit.

So, the question then arises: How to connect? If you connect in thought, you receive consciousness. And how should the connection be performed in order to receive Spirit? That is, creation means creation of all elements; you should know how to create your own spiritual basis. And then the technology of spiritual development will not be limited by some instantaneous or, for example, creative, impulse, or by reading, or by development of some, perhaps, specialized technologies. When you follow the main principle „thou shalt not kill, thou shalt not destroy“, then, as it happens, you have an infinite structure for development of the Spirit. And from that it follows that since there is a principle „do not destroy“ („thou shalt not destroy“ is how it sounds), in there, as soon as you built on the basis of all the existing elements your optimizing position, you instantly are transported into the structure of information creation. That is, here I have announced the overall fundamental principle, which has not been announced for a rather lengthy time, in view of the fact that there was no such problematic situation with respect to the possibility of global destruction; however, at this time, this principle must be announced. I am doing so for the first time. Here the meaning of this principle is as follows:

As soon as you are building without destroying anything, you come to the elements of creating any and all information, in fact, to the true knowledge of the Creator.

Therefore, this way you should be eternal not only because you, so to speak, are building, or want to do so, but this is the way you have been created, because true creation means eternity. Therefore, since you have been created as eternal, you must simply find the perspective of eternity in controlling the external and internal environment. How, for example, do you locate this perspective of eternity in each event? This is a special technology — and as I said — it is mastered by the experience of harmony of development, and in the future, as it happens, next year when you come, that is where I place the technology of non-destruction. That is, the technology, which states that you, using the harmonious constructive principle, can always regenerate yourself: first, by preventing the problem from occurring; and secondly, through complete restoration at any point in space-time.

Then at this point the following ideological principle is set:

Having an accomplished spiritual basis, you can create elements of development not only in the favorable environment that is already there, but you can enhance the environment.

That is, it actually says that if you have a direction of the creative development, then you should transfer this creativity onto any informational objects. The meaning here is that you can follow the creative path of development, and this is the only path, but this movement must be accompanied by the fact that for you there should be no limitations to that development. That is, in this case, you already support the structure of development in the status of the eternity of your creation.

That is, in this case, so that you would perform correctly a common event, for example, a healing of someone, or a simple regulation: optimization of an event, so that it would be done properly — that is, all this event must be of such a nature that it would exist always and everywhere (all this event means the entire complex). Once you reach this element, it means that your approach to resolving this task is technologically correct. From the standpoint of control in healing, this means to use this principle outlined here. You restore it in such a way that the organ actually is eternal, that is, and you immediately envisage all possible connections of this organ of this organism. Thus, you bring rules into its structure, which are set forth by the Creator. Rules mean what has been created initially, let's say, and towards where the human was directed.

That is, what we are talking about is that the Truth of the Creator, that is, what was bound by His Truth and what the Truth was and what was conveyed — it is that the Soul is eternal, and therefore the concept of eternity is transferred to the body as well. That is, as soon as we have this perspective, then there are no means for global destruction, and then it makes no sense to develop nuclear weapons. That is, it means that now has come such a time when the next element shall be an announcement regarding the eternity being of that element of the Soul, which is the body. That is, in this case, the Truth of the Creator starts developing into infinity, and that is what personifies the Creator himself. That is, actually the reverse development from the point of what has been accomplished, and this is the action of the Creator; therefore, naturally, control of the event may be performed based on the same principle. When you see movement from that which has been accomplished towards you, then you can change what has already been accomplished — this is control over the past. If you see what you would like to have, for example, in the future or the present, then reverse movement transitions into forward movement. That is, the existing principle can be simply transferred into forward movement. That is, the existing technology for control of the past can be transferred by doing as little as placing the thought in the future, and already you can control the past.

That is, by presenting what I am presenting here, I am showing that any technology can be converted into that very technology which you need. That is, the principle of instantaneous salvation is based on this. Actually, if you have once performed an action and received the result of optimization, that also tells you that you are saved and that you can save, and, to put it in an even more precise way — you will save yourselves and others. That is, in the technologies of salvation, you should use any logically completed, or spiritually, or soulfully accomplished structure in order to reinforce it positively in eternity.

Thus, the next stage is reinforcement of the elements that have been achieved and extending them into an eternal construct. That is, for example you have healed someone with one impulse, if you have restored a single cell, from that you can derive that you can; that you are eternal and can save others. That is actually the element of self-restoration and eternal existence, that is, non-destruction, is conditioned by the fact that not only are you coming from a spiritual structure, for example, but you are going towards a spiritual structure from the event. This way, by uniting those two statuses, it is naturally clear that you come even closer to the structure of your own Soul and organization of the body. That is, what I said already makes it possible to perform regeneration. But the matter in question is that in the course of detailed study and as you understand this technology deeper and deeper it becomes completely impossible to destroy you at all. That is, this is the basic ideology which you should be implementing. And what is another reason for implementing it? The ones working on the basis of this ideology, they pass the ideology to the next ones, etc., etc. And so it is that they are the ones providing true correct knowledge in the conditions when a system of global destruction is in existence. And since, after all, I am teaching to you specifically the system of salvation, this very context, the index, so to speak , of disseminating information around you in the form of thoughts, actions is a meaningful one, a matter of principle in all your subsequent actions.

So, by the next lecture it will be necessary to prepare this, so to speak, thought form, this kind of condition of the Spirit and Soul, in which you must convert to the eternal status, both that of your own and that of others, an element which is at a completely minimized stage, as it seems (that is, you are capable of sending an impulse, heal at least one cell, not even mentioning that you already capable of regulating events, of healing), but you must be able to transfer at least a minimal impulse of the restorative attribute. This is it actually: the system of salvation according to your, so to speak, level of development. The part that is special is that you can master this technology by simply listening, without even understanding, simply by taking this tape, and just by contemplating it. That is, in this system of salvation, access is implied via any of the possible channels. Or, for example, I have dictated it all, and even if you were not sitting here and listening, you would still be among the saved (this is what is called the „individual system of salvation“) and of course, save others.

So it means that by the next lecture it will be necessary to formalize the task, and make the minimal accomplished creative elements eternal.

Lecture 5

This lecture provides knowledge on how the spiritual basis reproduces events, and these events are a ready element of the impulse of the Spirit. That is, actually an event which is located outside space and time, which is an element of the impulse of that Spirit which created the event in question. That is, actually I am showing to you this system of connections when you have a variety of information, that is, all the connections, in each element of these connections.

So, you want to construct a certain situation, and you have it at the level of the Spirit (because you are taking it from somewhere). That is, actually when you want to construct a certain situation, heal someone, guide someone, or transform an event, you are taking the initial set: first, if you want to heal someone, there is a diagnosis; but if you want to make an event into something that you need, then to a significant extent you are frequently setting your own goals. So, when you set your own goals, you set them on the basis of known attributes, for example, the diagnosis or elements of events. And a part that is truly yours, that is, spiritual, coming from your Spirit, from your Soul, means that it is this element that is the main one from the standpoint of control, and this element serves to form the events which I mentioned. That is, the events which you are constructing already exist at the level of your Spirit.

Actually, having studied your own spiritual structure at the level of reproducing the completed, already known, pre-constructed events, you come to the level of the Soul. So the Spirit from this standpoint is a known factor for the Soul, that is, the Soul creates the event within the limits of the spiritual structure, and you receive these events for your consciousness. When you have considered this position of the World, you immediately see that the World exists on a spiritual basis, because this is precisely from where events emerge.

It turns out that in order to receive an event, you need to know in what way your spiritual basis creates them. Since I already talked about this, what one should do, but I purposely left out some connecting details; however, I did say and even repeated myself, stating that the spiritual basis makes them, and asked the question again: How? It is clear that it creates them at the point where the spiritual basis intersects, for example, the basis of the event. For example, if it is a material event — this is healing diseases, this is creation of the necessary event; if it is spiritual, that is, the sensory part (feelings, thoughts) — this is creation of the necessary thoughts, for example, the necessary feelings, etc.

There is an element which pertains to the feeling of Love, there are eternity and infinity present there. The system there is different, there is a system of sort of absolute statics — this is different and pertains not only to the spiritual basis, but also the basis of the Soul, the basis of the World. Therefore, Love is considered — and it actually is — the basis which possesses both infinite and local factors. When you consider this stage you see that the World is created out of Love. That is, it is sufficient to realize that, and you create on the basis of Love, that is, meaning that Love is the building block of any event.

When you build one building block, a second, and third one, the result is the Spirit. The Spirit is a reflection of Love from the standpoint of recreation of events. It is the word „Love“ that describes this technologically, for example. When you view it neutrally, that is, without words, then you have the Spirit; but when you want to obtain the technology, you will examine the first position from the standpoint of Love. The word „creation“ gives the overall picture, and it is frequently vague, and Love is the building block of any event. So, when they say that the Creator-God has created and His creations are such that He shows Love towards them, this is the way it is, simply based on the technology of how the World is set up.

So, by analogy with how the Creator created, you act accordingly. Having reviewed the element presented as Love, you look at how the connections are being set up between the elements of the structure, and then you transfer it to other structures — to perception in the form of some feelings, creative feelings, feelings of desire to build something, etc., and then you watch how the transfer of the concept of Love is going on in transformation of the word. That is, when you do it, you must also understand, you can understand, how will it be transformed, for example, into words. That is, here it is important to receive this technology of development of one's own Spirit so that the words are the components of this Spirit, of this state of the Spirit. That is, when you have a state, you have words, and the words are already being built. That is why there is such a principle stating that „in the beginning there was the word".

When you examine the verbal phase, that is, the descriptive phase, you can instantaneously abstract away from it and obtain the non-verbal phase — the phase which was not described, but where everything is known. This is the state of the Spirit, it also exists. You are not even, for example, looking there; the events are seemingly far away, but you know about them. There is an example in physics: it is ascribed to Lomonosov, I think: if somewhere far away there is a forest, you cannot see the trees moving, but when you come close you can see it is an optical principle. But nonetheless, somewhere far away you know that there is a forest there, that it is there specifically, but you do not want to come close, for example. Then it happens that on the spiritual basis, and that is what I am getting at, it is always known what is ahead. And your task is to simply take it from there. And when you take it, for example, and often if you have to take it from one construct only, then what you receive is precisely the system of salvation, and you receive it so that you, naturally, can offer salvation, because you frequently follow the only possible path, where no other options are possible. From this follows precise diagnostics, precise control, etc.

Therefore, your task in all of this will be to understand this lecture from the standpoint of your own Spirit, and see how your Soul organizes this Spirit at the time of understanding this lecture. This will do for now; later, in about a month and a half, you have to make an appointment for a meeting and come with your results.

Control for the Purpose of Improving Health

April 18, 2002

Good afternoon. During today's meeting I will tell you about the methods of effecting control through the structure of your own consciousness based on your specific requests. Today we shall work in the following way: initially, I will present sort of an overview in the form of a lecture, i.e., I will show the following methods of control via the structure of the consciousness, and in doing so it is necessary to take into account that it will pertain only to the specific requests, which have been given here. Secondly, we will summarize the information with respect to a specific future situation, which is no longer related to this request.

I will be working on the requests from 10:00 pm to 11:00 pm for three days.

All the action that is associated with today‘s action will be divided into the following: I first will present the material in the form of a lecture, that is, I will provide the methodology for working with specific tasks. This methodology extends to other actions by the transferring such universal systems, about which I will speak.

From the standpoint of structuring the consciousness in accordance with my system of salvation and harmonious development, it is thus necessary to isolate in the perception the controlling optical level in such a way that the control itself is such that the spheres which you perceive as optical spheres are informed. And therefore, since it is necessary to use the simplest possible systems for control, it is necessary here to demonstrate the functions of targeted direction of your actions in accordance with the system of general interconnections.

According to this system, it is necessary, above all, that there is no possible global destruction and there is implementation of the technology of harmonious development.

In this regard, control put this way, in fact, is rather simple from the standpoint of the elements of perception and runs up against only the fact that you must isolate in your perception precisely that kind of sphere of macro-regulation, where you ensure namely the first level — i.e., a possible global catastrophe does not occur, and you actually ensure the next level of control, i.e., in the next second you can perform some actions, since the catastrophe did not occur.

In this case, the element of harmonious development is ensured and set forth, and performance of specific tasks is also ensured.

Consequently, my system of control (according to the system of salvation and harmonious development), in this case, lies in the fact that you isolate in perception by different methods first the macrosphere, and then sort of a special sphere, establish a connection in such a way that your special event occurs simultaneously as you are accomplishing namely this macro-regulation. That is, you do not allow for the possibility of a global catastrophe and ensure harmonious development.

In order to do this technologically, that is, use nothing but the elements of the consciousness, some elements need to be used that are sufficiently accessible from the standpoint of your previous experience of performing any actions.

Now I propose to examine four methods for implementing this technology.

First method: using concentration on numbers.

Second method: using concentration on letters, i.e., words.

Third method: concentration on colors.

Fourth method: concentration on sounds and shapes.

This is sufficiently accessible technology and, most importantly, it is generally acceptable in terms of how well it is known, i.e., all these things are fairly well-known and you have already used them many times.

Therefore, in this case, first of all, we need to consider the model of perception in relation to what you want, for example, to implement for yourself. This is the so-called perception model; the point of it is that you, above all, must see a certain optical signal in your perception and single out, at the very beginning, the sphere of macro-regulation.

The concept of an optical signal — this is, generally speaking, a rather simple concept, but in some cases it needs to be singled out.

So, it is necessary to work on singling out this signal, first of all, at the beginning of the technology that uses concentration, as I mentioned, on numbers, words (letters), color, sound and shape.

And it is namely this singling out works as follows: if you, for example, are looking at some image, then it is possible to visualize that image; that is, the primary optical component is already present in perception.

The element of singling out the optical signal, the one containing the sphere of macro-regulation, is that you can view any physical object as if it were located as close in front of you as possible; for example, I can look at a dictaphone as physical and imagine a dictaphone while doing so.

And so the connection of the physical level, which is perceived by vision, and the dictaphone, which I imagine, as if overlapping the two images, at a point as close as possible to me, to the physical body, the sphere of macro-regulation is singled out.

That is, this method of singling out this sphere is sort of in an automatic mode, when you form it from the dynamics, from the action.

Why does it happen this way? Because if in the visualization I impose what

I am imagining onto the logically existing dictaphone in physical perception, therefore the element of reality did exist; therefore it was ensured that there was no macrodestruction. And hence the sphere itself is singled out.

This is the first method, which in the future already leads to the fact that your specific tasks, they proceed from the fact that they are inside this sphere or are a result of the development of this sphere. And so if you view the element of control as the result and as a development of this sphere, then in control via the number, in the number itself this very attribute needs to be considered. That is, the numbers which ensure control of the result, that is, control over your specific event.

Your specific event may be healing, your own self-regeneration, or treatment of any other person, or maybe it is not a person, but a plant, an animal, etc., control of any system of reality.

Therefore, the concept of particular events is a rather broad concept; the most important thing here is to immediately narrow it down for your specific goal.

Thus, by performing this control, you immediately take part in the system of ensuring macro-safety and thereby ensure the most concentrated flow of information, which ensures completion of your tasks, and you accomplish the specific mission for implementing a system of global security.

Therefore, here it is necessary to understand that the concentration of information for this control specifically occurs because you are working through the macro-level.

Thus, having singled out this sphere by superimposing two elements in perception and what is perceived by vision, you are already working, in fact, in the best way, if this action of yours is a consequence of the macrosphere, within this sphere, i.e., the boundary conditions are sufficiently clear to you.

The sphere itself is silvery-white, not very large in diameter.

You sort of mentally enter this sphere. And then you work by numbers, i.e., singling out the control-number involves the following: the sphere itself is designated by the "one"; the number for the action itself is number "two", which is the center of the sphere, and it is necessary to include in this action the meaning of your control, what it is that you want. If this is healing from osteochondrosis, then you must formulate this information and either examine the presumed area of the spine, or you must state it in words and insert it in the center of the sphere and designate it simply by the number "two".

So, control lies merely in the fact that you isolate within the sphere between the center and sort of the external surface — this is number "one"; you designate, for example, number "three" or "four" that is, the next number, which is arranged due to the fact that you concentrate both at the center of the sphere and on the sphere itself.

And the technology is in fact very simple. With some practice you will start to find the place where this number "three" or "four" manifests itself in your perception. Besides, it fixates rather specifically in one and the same place; and your task is simply to concentrate on one number, and this is number "three" or "four". Why "four"? This is a method of summarizing information, just in case, we take into account some external nuances of reality. In fact for the most part the matter in question is concentration on the number "three"; for example, in the course of healing osteochondrosis, the number "three" is located on the radius between the center of the sphere, macro-regulation, and its sort of internal surface, and on the radius which is directed specifically towards us, that is, towards your physical body. And it often happens that it is the point closest to the physical body.

If, for example, it is a question of curing diabetes mellitus, then the vector is directed in the opposite direction, and the number "three" is located on that radius, which is directed sort of the other way, in the direction opposite from you.

It is sufficient just to proceed mentally along the radius, and you can set, in principle, that point as the point of resistance to the movement of thought. Then you can simply concentrate in this place and treat, in this way, the diabetes mellitus, and in principle work with any situation.

Thus, concentration on numbers, it is very simple in this case and involves you yourself isolating the number.

As soon as you know how to isolate the number, then formulating the problem and bringing it forth into the center, this is not a very difficult task; simply imagine it as the central point or a small sphere. Then isolating the number "three" is just a task to practice working with this macrosphere.

The second principle is working with words, i.e., the principle of this type of control is that in fact you are working with letters. Since any words can be used, it is sufficient to isolate the controlling system in letters, and isolating in letters does not different much from that for numbers. In this case, it is necessary to simply isolate the sphere, again macro-regulation, as much as possible according to a principle which is close to the principle used for numbers. The only difference is that in numbers, it is a more discrete system, i.e., the purpose of control has to be stated; it is better to state any objective in the form of words, and it is better if it is not an exceedingly lengthy statement. Then you take the resulting text and memorize it — at least in the form of images, at least some part of the text... and you have to do it twice: once in a spatial location next to yourself and in another one sort of nearby. And so you do not have to write it down — it is sufficient to formulate it. Just obtain two images of the same text. However, it is best to combine the text in a specific point in front of you; in other words, it is better to work in physical space in front of you so that you will have stability in work. It reinforces the same effect.

The macro-regulation sphere is isolated, i.e., it is done very simply, using the following simple technological procedure: let's say I have the sheet with the request. I can visualize it in the consciousness and can imagine it, for example, in a location above the sheet, or at a level next to the sheet. And mentally combining them, for example, on the same physical sheet (I can, in principle, work on the same physical sheet, that is, sort of through the system of visualization); then the lower left border of the sheet, if this is a planar system, isolates the macro-regulation sphere. So in this case the principle is the same: isolating the sphere is the action. So here is the logical status, and it is clear in the sense that the verbal phase virtually does not change when it is transferred onto the sheet; thus, working with the visualization is the same as working with physical space.

Therefore, having completed the procedure for isolating it, we have the result that the sphere is already here, and there is no need to search, no need to use up time or to concentrate on looking for this sphere.

Lower left border — this sphere is already ready. Further, the principle is similar: you take the text, sort of archive the sphere, or you can simply put it (the text) inside, into the center of this sphere of macro-regulation, and further actions are already a special technology. You continue to work after all these actions. You are working, it turns out, in the lower left corner of the sheet. You work in such a way that the letters are collected from the text in order to have the top part in a symmetrical pattern; I can sort of take and divide the letters symmetrically into two mechanical parts — this is the information of macro-regulation, macro-salvation, and the lower one — this is what corresponds to your particular task. As informing two parts: the upper one is the macro-regulation of the text, simply informing the text, and the lower part informs that this is the solution for your task. You receive a controlling effect, you receive the solution for the task which is stated in this text.

By the way, here you can apply the principle of the same number: you can do it between the sphere itself and the center of the central sphere, within which control occurs; you can also, for example, concentrate on the number between the two spheres. By this concentration you simply enhance the effect. You can obtain the number by the same method, about which I spoke at the time of concentration on the number.

The point is that in this case the principle is in fact very simple when you listen to it for a bit. Speech just comes down to the fact that, in the end, you take the recorded text and divide it into two parts, as if using a ruler: the top and the bottom, roughly symmetrically, but it does not have to be precise. In the upper part, you place the information for macro-regulation; you simply consider that on the top — this is just the physical part of the text, which corresponds to information of macro-regulation, and on the bottom — this is what corresponds to your particular problem.

And by performing a number of those concentrations along the text, simply on the physical sheet, by performing the concentration specifically in this place, i.e., inside this sphere, i.e., you must visualize the technology, you receive the effect of control, perform control with respect to the task of the text.

The third level of control is through colors.

When we say: control through color, above all, it is clear that the concept of color is a rather comprehensive or infinite presentation of the concept: until we apply the color to some surface, we perceive the color as an infinite system, i.e., this is like the information of the color.

And so, in this case, working with color is meant specifically as working with information of the color, that is, there is some primary action, some primary basis, information, which the color sort of contains, that is, some color background. Therefore, working with color is subdivided into fairly simple working in this context. You isolate at the level of thought namely the background of this color; it can be compared to an unripe nut, where your information regarding the goal is contained inside, and you are just taking off the outer shell of the nut. So here is the only point: the sphere of macro-control is obviously located inside together with the objective of your control. That is, here you do not divide the work with color: the objective of control and the sphere of macro-regulation. Furthermore, you have access, above all, in the fact that when you begin working, you must know immediately that you will not be dividing, first of all, the sphere of macro-regulation with the sphere of your tasks. This is as if one, internal information of light and color, lies on this surface of the sphere.

Your task in terms of control is to make sure that you take the light of the necessary color and sort of mentally disconnect it from this sphere and sort of make it infinite. That is the very meaning of this control.

In order to know which color to choose, here one can use a fairly simple principle for finding a color for a specific task. So, the principle of finding the color is as follows: let's take a specific practical example here. Let us assume it is necessary to cure angina pectoris, then I concentrate in the center of the isolated sphere. You must make sure to pay attention here because I designate all these actions. I do not use a sheet of paper; I do not use physical space: I am working only within the limits of my own perception. The difference is fundamental, the work in physical perception, namely in perception, still may be in physical space as well, but it is namely perception. I can perceive the physical space of a table, for example, but the space of perception may be not located here, i.e., in principle it is possible to imagine that I can perceive something in any point in this room or in any point in reality.

That is, bear in mind that the space of perception is a different space (in this case).

Why am I presenting different systems in this case? Because when you are just working in practice, or using one method or another, it happens not infrequently that, for example, you do not have a concept at hand that you have a table or that you can use written text; therefore, for those cases when you need to exert control quickly and use some system, which would delay you, it is better to use control via color. Usually this happens in those cases when you are facing a complex problem, for example, with angina pectoris, which can lead to a heart attack, then it is better to work through color. Therefore, here, as soon as you concentrate on the task of isolating the color namely in the center of the sphere, then the light begins to turn into optical light, in such a way that it begins to acquire color, and you will see the color which is the controlling color with respect to this system.

That is, the control task comes down to isolating this light. And why is the sphere of macro-regulation united with the sphere of your specific tasks? Because the color as an infinite system in the structure of consciousness does not provide strict borders in terms of differentiation. Therefore, in this case macro-regulation is combined with the sphere of your control. When you concentrate in the center of, let's say, of this nut, then it is possible, let us assume, to select any element, but it is better to select something close, for example, to start working using familiar images (nut, onion) using some very well-known elements, where it is possible to take the "skin" off, let's put it that way. And when you visualize at first this element in optical space, then work in the center of this element is sufficiently clear to you; it is quite clear where the center is of some fruit or vegetable.

As soon as you start working with specific examples, still you should consistently move towards working with images. It is better not to work for a long time with specific elements of reality, physical ones, because in this case the matter in question is that in accordance with the system of salvation it is frequently necessary to use superfast access to information, for example, so that some catastrophic event does not occur.

And if you get used to working with an image, then you will spend time in order to generate an image; it is better for you to work with an image which does not belong to physical reality, but simply form this sphere mentally, concentrate in the center, and so the first color that starts to gather — for example, for curing angina pectoris — it will be a hue of violet color in this case.

You take and sort of using a mental effort, in the planar view, remove some sort of film from the surface of this sphere, remove it until this color comes off the surface of this sphere and it disperses. During this, in the work space the coloration becomes light violet, that is, the light becomes more diluted, and gradually only some tinges of this color remain. If you still can perceive the signs at this stage, it is better to do it again, until you see, for example, this same sphere turn white or silvery white; that is, you must work, while even the minimal tinges of color remain.

The logical principle of this control is: you actually make the information of the objective infinite, because color is an infinite value in the consciousness. As soon as you isolate an element of color from some overall volume, considering that this color is the solution for your problem, you send an infinite distribution of your task, and the controlling action is performed through the system of general connections. That is in this case a significant amount is done with the help of the constructive forces which participate in this process.

The principle is very simple, that you only have to announce something, and the information comes, it will be realized, reaction to physical realities occurs, i.e., for example, the cure or some physical event. In doing so, you are also participating in macro-regulation, i.e., ensuring macro-creation.

The fourth principle of control: control through sound and shape.

The work is very simple here, for example, with respect to what I just said. There are some extremely simple aspects of this work, but still here it is important to see that the concepts of simplicity in work with certain elements of perception are different in the sense that even though the level appears simple, it is frequently situated on a very highly-charged next level.

And so if you are working using simple coordinates, you may encounter strong resistance or development of the level, where you frequently have to use deep control in a discrete manner, i.e., non-trivial methods.

Therefore, this is the way to consider the concept of simplicity in this case. And the explanation here is as follows: if we review, for example, the concept of shape, that is control via shapes, in principle, or control via sound or sound shape, then in perception it is possible to see the shape of sound and at the same time hear this sound, for example, at the level of perception.

Organization of shape or organization of the sort of pre-sound system — this is that system which can be organized prior to the beginning of the optical element of perception.

That is, a shape can be organized as an element of reality, but in doing so the shape may change, which is understandable. That is, it is possible to assemble some object from the elements of an erector set, but the erector set elements themselves can be perceived in perception as, for example, a pre-element level. This is because we work in the consciousness through some elemental level, i.e., this is either a number, a word or a color.

And if we want to pose the question of how in general to initially assemble the color that was there, let us assume, before the color? Then we will be able to work with a comparable concept, let us assume, sound, which is organized by vibrations, let us assume, of the structure of light. Further, naturally, either we can consider that through shape we organize sound or color. Work with shape is rather simple, because this is a level which is located before the level of optically densely manifested information. But in doing so, if we want to work through the structures, let us assume, of shape, then here we need a connection with a sort of correlating system; in this case, it may be sound, i.e., a vector system, directing the objective of control of the shape.

The principle is very simple. If you take a magnet and small particles of iron, let's say, and scatter them, when the magnet is brought close to these small particles, they will all start moving in the direction of the magnet.

That is, the shapes must be controllable immediately. Therefore, in this case, I am showing control of shape and sound at the same time, where shape is the system of organizing the sound system of perception.

For control in this case it is sufficient to put in the shape of a sphere the fact that macro-destruction does not occur under any combinations of the events of eternal, harmonious development, plus there is still the solution for your personal task. That is, as if into one shape — this can be any shape, let‘s assume, a sphere or that which you identify as your own shape. That is, here it is important to identify the individual shape of control, if in the future you are going to develop namely this sound and shape system.

When you have identified this shape, it is important to consider which sound, from your point of view, is the controlling sound with respect to this shape.

And in fact it is a very simple characteristic. You sort of start training and begin hearing the sound as soon as you see the control shape, i.e., you simply isolate it from three sorts of simultaneous compositions.

Then the control task is just to maintain by concentration the intensity of this sound.

Let us assume that the mantra principle of control lies in the fact that mantras organize one — low or high —concentration sound, and this is maintained for some time.

In this case, you simply do not work verbally, but work just through the structure of perception, but in principle you do perform extraneous actions. But what is more, in this case you can, unlike in certain systems of generalized mantras, you can create completely specific control, which you place in the center of this or some other limited shape.

Thus, again, as I said, the principle is very simple: you are working here even before the beginning the optical level of perceiving information.

But to assemble the shape, that is, hold it in a structure where there is no information, that is, you have sort of nothing to “latch” onto, nothing that would have the consciousness oriented and therefore there is, not even on this plane, a closer concept, that you do not even have a space in order to work. And when there is no external space, if there is no optical shape, there is no level around which you need to work. That is, if you work with numbers, with letters or color, then at least you have that color, letter, or number, or any other image of perception.

In this case, your task is to form and therefore, on the one hand, simplicity of control, it may not even be described by some word, because the word is formed after there is an identified component, if only a letter. And therefore, this is sort of a pre-word level of control; it can be most effective, and therefore here we must understand that work in seemingly simple coordinates in fact may be, on the contrary, a system more complex in principle. The most important thing here is to maintain the shape in the space of perception.

As soon as you learn to maintain this shape in practice, then in principle there are no major problems, and there are certain methods of control over the thought-shape which develops in photonic conditions, or a type of camera, like a video camera, which register the thought as, for example, a photon beam.

And if in this case we view from the standpoint of this video camera how thinking occurs, which organizes control through shapes, it can be seen there very clearly that there is sort of a center of organization of the world; if you take information from all of the world, for example, and consider that this is optical information of some sphere, then the center of organization of this information and the center of thought for us will immediately start coming in alignment in this way of work. Because you come to the level of organization of information and, accordingly, this level, of course, frequently requires work with many parameters and in many directions. Therefore, in this case, formulation of words, formulation of some objectives of control — frequently this is already a cause-and-effect system. And here to a more significant extent the spiritual system of control is implemented, where you can work without formulating words or images, but simply after exerting logical control to attain at a spiritual level, a state which means control on the basis of the spiritual aspect, and then you have it, that this action is performed due to a particular state of the spirit.

Then it turns out that this state is also control. Here you very quickly need to train the system of control through development of a distinctive king of training and remember the spiritual state in the control systems.

And in the future this spiritual state is universal, if we are talking about you attaining a system for curing some specific single disease, then only in the given spiritual state and concentration of the spirit at a specific point, you achieve, first of all, a cure from this specific disease. But at the same time, according to the attribute of dissemination, self-development of creative systems, it is possible to cure other diseases as well by sort of differentiating the spiritual state.

Therefore, when through the logical phases of control you transition to control namely through the state of the spirit, through a state beyond the soul, then control in the future — this is already a rather calm phase of your development. Here, performing some everyday task or while not exerting active control, you can in fact be an active controlling entity, since your memory and your spirit are working namely according to the most optimal systems, which you obtained from the logical phase.

As homework, to the extent possible, try to transform the logical element, which I have described, which is work with the logical phase of perception — these are numbers, words, letters, colors or sound — transform, for example, into the level of work namely through the work of the spirit. And then you will see that here there is a universal principle of dissemination of information, and very quickly it will begin to engage. That is, if you ask the question of how to transform the cure of a particular type of diabetes mellitus, for example, into curing some other system or some other disease, specifically identified, that is in the treatment there may be a system of the organism. But it can, for example, be considered a normal condition at this time, that is, there are very fine transitions here. Therefore, let's assume that it is a question of curing, which will record the normal status at any diagnostic level. Then it turns out that development of this system is best done through accessing namely the system of spiritual concentrations.

Then you receive a sufficiently stable form of control, which in principle is nothing more than the state of the spirit at a given moment with respect to the given task.

And when you examine this aspect, then, if you transfer back to the optical, the so-called logical principle of control, it is sufficiently clear why it happens this way.

The spiritual structure is similar to a high concentration of light; if we want to normalize, for example, some process which is reflected in the logical phase, it will suffice for us to move that light there, and a high concentration of light resolves sort of a series of issues, unlike the local levels of the logical phase of control.

Therefore, one can use synthesis in control here, although this is not an objective in itself — namely to work just on the spiritual phase of control.

Consequently, if the logical level of control is something you are better at, then work on the logical basis. But as for the summarization phase, that is, for example, in this case I tied the control to the specific tasks, which are stated now either in the form of a request, or if someone is mentally stating the task at today's meeting with the purpose of control for his specific task, then further on, the second level, this is who is listening to the lecture, can resolve their tasks — this is sort of the second optical ring.

And the third task — this is to create the universalism of such a plane so that those who perceive it could pass on this technology to others and so that in the future, without diminishing the optical level of the intensity of the shining, it would be passed on infinitely, with the purpose of developing the kind of structure of consciousness which can self-regenerate the organism or build its own structure of consciousness or external reality.

Therefore, the level of generalization, in order to send it into a very distant time, it is better to work on the spiritual aspect, when there is the principle of transfer — it is also infinite. If I need to transmit on a specific level, for example, to the present time, then I can bring it into the logical phase and transmit it on specifically, perhaps at the targeted level; if it is for physicians, the next element of the transmission needs to be such that the physicians would understand it; if it is for children or construction workers, then, respectively, it can be transmitted to them; whoever knows something specifically, you need to use their level of knowledge.

If it is for children, it is better to transmit bearing in mind ensuring the required development for children, that is, taking into account the tasks of intensity of development of the children.

That is, insofar as possible, as independent work look at the levels of transmission of control information in the macro-salvation system of consciousness, and in precisely this way that during technology transfer it would be transferred with the same intensity as when, for example, you listened and understood.

The task of this transfer may also frequently be achieved rather quickly at the level of the state of the spirit, because the condition of the spirit is transmitted within the level of training and control rather easily and quickly. And you have perhaps noticed, when studying in different systems, including school, that if a teacher, while explaining his subject, was in some state or other then it was possible to see at the ordinary physical level, how much more intensive the knowledge transfer was when you see a familiar state.

This is the principle of recognition, the principle of the so-called familiar state, related to the rather specific technology of macro-access. In fact, this is the technology of access into any system of control; that is, it is possible to stop an explosion of a nuclear reactor; it is possible, if a plane is falling, to materialize a circuit board or restore the consciousness of the pilot. In my practice there were cases when pilots had poisoning, and there all that could be done, since the cabin was locked, was to restore their consciousness, and it was restored successfully. Here it is important to see yet another principle, that in the conditions of technogenic development, sufficient control of external systems is the way that is already necessary now to a significant extent. And in the future, during techno-cybernetization of society, it will become the only possible option altogether, when it will be possible to monitor the movement of external systems simply by the fact that you will be able to control them. And, by the way, I am making in this regard a system of specific crystals which would capture the thought and generate the controlling impulse, for example, to the technical systems.

All the same, technical advancements in the future will be such as to take into consideration, above all, that technical equipment should not destroy humans. For this you must, using your consciousness, be able to determine the precise coordinates of the technical system and, for example, indicate the trajectory of development of this system.

So, on the whole, that is what I wanted to say at today's meeting on technologies of control, related to specific tasks of today, because, as a rule, the tasks presented largely shape the chosen ideology, the methodology of the material that I present. The task, I believe, insofar as possible, your task is to make sure that this material can be disseminated, that is, it is desirable that you make yourself fluent in it so that already after the initial levels, which you have heard about during the meeting, you start disseminating the technology immediately and immediately receive, best of all, the elements of control. There is no need to separate, for example, the phases of learning from the phase of action, because in the technology of salvation frequently even the minimal amount of information is such that it needs to be used immediately for control, for obtaining specific results.

Therefore, to the extent possible, monitor what is most important — the result, the result at the informational level, that is, you perceive some problem and shed light on it. And the second option is when you have some task, when you have it at the physical level, you work on this task and track it as correctly as possible how it was implemented in detail, maybe in general, and what were the results at a specific time.

That is, when you practice constantly, the control system will become ever more concentrated for you and increasingly simpler and clearer. In a certain sense, it will be the normal state, which makes it possible to resolve at least this one issue, that there will not be a possible global catastrophe, for sure, and in addition to resolve in parallel a specific task in the direction of eternal development.

Therefore, I believe that this meeting should be held so that even listening to what you perceived as a number of separate elements, it is better to accept at once with respect to your specific tasks.

In addition to the fact that I will be working on my own specific tasks from 10:00 pm to 11:00 pm for three days, today, tomorrow and the day after tomorrow, on requests using control, but in this control I will place a significant part on the further transfer of knowledge on today‘s meeting. To the maximum extent possible, intensively use, first of all, the phrase, as I said, that which you have now, plus that which you will have, for example, in the form of a dictaphone recording, etc.

You can use some of my materials from previous lectures.

But on the whole, this competes our today's meeting.

Thank you for your attention. All the best to you. Good-bye.

Teaching on Salvation and Harmonious Development

Action with the Body of the One God

April 18, 2003

Hello.

The topic of today's seminar is the implementation and dissemination of the „Teaching on Salvation and Harmonious Development", using the method — „Action with the Body of the One God „. What we are saying is, that when we talk about the body of God, the action is determined, firstly, by our own essence; that is, we act, because we have a body, and the body is a creation of God. Therefore, when we act together with the body, we imply that we also see the external controlling image on the part of God. Therefore in this method, first and foremost, it is necessary to determine the speed of action; that is, by determining the speed characteristics of action, we come to the logic of understanding how this action is defined from the standpoint of attaining the result. In normal practice it is logically clear for people that the issue of speed is always related to how we go over the options in order to achieve a certain result. That is, speed is an organic function stemming from the essence of a biological organism. Therefore, when you perform an action, the organism works in a way; it is, generally speaking, involved at a non-breakable level in the system of action: it is the external reality, internal feelings and some logical considerations or clairvoyant outlines.

In connection with this, it is possible to consider the manifestation of the body of God, the physical body of God, as an element, which is determined, generally speaking, by the totality of events. In addition, when we talk about physics as if about nature, some external environment, then being the body of the One God, It should be constructed in accordance with the image which is the same as the Soul in the image of God, and the human body — in the image of God. That is, here sort of the reverse principle is used, but not quite; I did not mention it here that „in action" — is identical, absolutely precise. Because if we look at this simple principle: a ray of the sun is reflecting from something, for example, a piece of glass; the glass reflects this light towards the optics of perception, that is, towards a human eye. So then the manifestation of God here is expressed originally by the Sun; assuming earlier beliefs — this is, for example, the Sun. When a thought moves organically towards the original source, sort of closes on it, we are talking about manifestation, specifically about the physical level, where God is manifested physically.

So it is possible to see the One God closely, specifically in the physical body; it is possible simply by looking at some object of reality, having specified the cause and consequence at the same time. That is, by understanding both the essence of an object and its original existence, the same way as the ray coming from the sun. Where did that object come from altogether, what is its essence from the standpoint of God? That is, an appeal to God repeats two or more times. If we consider prayer — and many people, when praying, see God next to them, and, in addition to that, in the physical body — then the effect of the prayer is determined specifically by high-speed transfer of information, that is, the information exchange is very rapid. Because God, as a multilevel, in general, status of a personality, is defined by the fact that we see him, while at the same time very quickly doing something. I suppose that everyone has noticed that when things are happening very rapidly, particularly if those are extreme situations, the presence of God is simply there in the heart of a person, it is felt specifically as a creation of God; and many at such a moment plead with God for help. Therefore velocity characteristics with respect to control over the events — and this is a somewhat more complicated transition — including the speed of the events themselves, plus sort of integration with at least one of the levels of awareness, for example with the heart — all this is the consciousness of God, who has a physical body. That is, we see awakening of consciousness here as something that we are engaged in.

So it becomes apparent that God sent people to the elements of His own consciousness, which is from its inception eternal, that is, it includes all the elements of reality and all events. But at the same time it is a subject for the occupation of man, and man was created by God. Therefore it comes to the fact that such an enclosed autonomous system as God, who created everything, has a physical body. In that, this system coincides with the fact that the subject of analysis is an element either static or developing through actions of men. Because a man studies the Consciousness of God and, at the same moment, (this is of tremendous applied importance) this element of action. Because, by understanding Consciousness, he comes to an understanding of how the physical body of God is set up. In general it is set up by analogy, of course, God, is, naturally — a man, maximally ideal in a certain sense, even though the concept of ideal in a large number of events is a rather conditional concept.

Because a person must be reactive like a normal person; form follows that action together with the body of the One God is the same action as an action with the body of man as the first postulate. And when you look at this as if at the level of comparison: it is possible, for example, to run somewhere with a person, do something, accomplish some tasks with a group of people or all people at once. So in accordance with my „Teaching on Salvation and Harmonious Development", the level for transferring information that goes directly from one person to everybody can be instantaneous — the same way as the One God transmits everything to everywhere at once for salvation of all And why is this attainable? Because it is clear that if we act together with the body, the physical body of the One God, then in practice we receive a very simple picture: do what He does, for instance, and that's all.

As for analogy and connection — that means looking at the way the body of one person interacts with the body of another person, how they act together, for example, playing ball or volleyball. So there is that optical light, that travels from person to person, is organized by God Himself, the One God. Then the way it works is the connection through a concatenation of events, which is present through all of this, and this light that travels from person to person — this is the light of the Soul, exclusively of the Soul only. A person shines on another person at the time of action only through the Soul. So there appears an element of action, this is what I mean by that, if you act with the body of God in accordance with the topic and method of today's lecture.

Of course, he can shine using the consciousness and other elements. But then when the question comes up that we always mean that there is an instructor, that it is necessary to act together with the body of God — we shine using only the Soul. So here is an element of the rigid structure of the World. The World is frequently structured so unequivocally rigidly at the level of information that physical manifestation is a very remote consequence. That is, the setup at the informational level of perception is more rigid and more fundamental. That is, there are laws present which may be unchanging altogether.

And in accordance with that we are coming closer to the fact that the person comes into the set of those laws that the reality of that level, it does not change. The light of the Soul and the Soul are eternal, and therefore the mutual shining, even one act of shining is eternal as well. Therefore, if we are saying that it is necessary to grow organs or be cured from a disease, then it is sufficient to sort of place the matrix of the person over that level where there are actions of God, but in the physical body. The technology is somewhat more complex, but in terms of simple understanding, it is as follows: if you consider such concepts as the body of God, which can be visualized and touched by people, who are created by God himself, that very sensation of a person; if you analyze the logical level of consciousness, then the sensation is that action, which is given originally is still in the action of God Himself. That is, God has to, at first, sort of touch, in the logic of human perception, and then exert control.

And so, in order to talk about such a concept as the physical body of God, specifically the One God, first and foremost, it is necessary to consider what comprises the action of the man himself, which (action) so far is only approaching the body of the physical level of God. If, for example, physically God is nearby, and man can act with him as just a person, the result has been achieved. But since the One God has the attributes of the individual, that is, He is located in one specific place at a specific time, then it means the action is with him, and he initially sets all actions. That is, generally this exists already all by itself: each physically acting person acts together with the physical body of God, because the element of the body is initially created by God; this is the logical link. So what we have here is the principle of simple approximation, approaching to that if even man does not physically see the One God, but it still works that way, that he can act together with him, which means to act correctly.

And the body of the One God is still an invincible construct: God cannot be destroyed, He cannot die, etc. And therefore, if you learn the principle of remote action level together with the body of God, that is, we are talking about action in general. Then it comes to the point that it is sufficient to master more or less precisely at least one action, even remote. But if the physical body of God is nearby, it is even better. So then we can transfer this attribute of action using the logical method. If somewhere very far away there is a forest, and we cannot see, using physical vision, the movement of every leaf, we can think logically and enter the microstructure if we know the internal design of a leaf. So entering the microstructure provides the knowledge that is actually a forest.

This is the diagnostics: that in fact there is a forest in the distance. So, here the crux of the matter is that we have, in essence, an understanding via a different diagnostic method, which is originally set up as a clairvoyance method, that this is actually foliage. That is, this is a higher level of development, such as the development of access through action — let's put it that way — such as a clairvoyance element of viewing. It provides the identification of the forest itself, that it is actually a person seeing a forest, specific kinds of trees, for example, based on the morphology of the leaves. So the applied meaning is: to see in perception the physical body of God. And in general, it is simply like the physical body of man. We can create an additional impulse here, which would be that we must enter some kind of parallel diagnostic channel as it was, for example, in the leaves, in morphology.

But then a very simple question arises, to which the answer is immediately available: that very simple element is actually the body of man. That is, since it is a creation of God, it is also a parallel, additional channel and therefore having studied this body on at least one level of action, there is no need to enter morphology, but to study action — why was there the action of the finger— and, when we realize that, we see, in essence, the action with God. We see the following: that the level of universal development is specifically aimed at having people act together with the body of God, including the physical one. Because they have been initially created by God, and therefore it follows from this logic that they already act on His behalf. And since He provided a physical body, then He must have designed the way it should move in different situational systems.

And with this the sign of the complete freedom of will of the individual is that from development towards God, that is, sort of remote access, works exactly in such a way so as to achieve non-destruction of the physical body — this is, first and foremost, the social norm. Why is it, for example, the systems of international law are directing us towards the normal social level? Because of the social mechanism: it is specifically peacefulness, a normal way of life without, for example, aggressive wars; this is a manifestation of an already more generic status, when physical bodies receive complete freedom of will. And then the way it works is that we have, practically, the kind of control that if we want to achieve, let's suppose, a complete cure of the gravest diseases, then this cure is simply normalizing the situation for the person and it can occur only because he can, in his social status, achieve a sort of regulation of the norm of life, where there are no wars, find a niche, which is free for him like dome kind of matrix system, in the course of reflecting onto which he is restored. That is, social laws represent a way to normalize and continue, and therefore man must reproduce the social systems in the same way as God. He should not destroy them in essence.

And if he, for example, is acting in this way then the body of the One God, manifested initially in man simply, and subsequently, man is at different times a creation of God; any man; and therefore his actions can be rendered at the infinite level absolutely safe. That is, technical advancements may be not at all harmful to people, and it can have, in principle, the same range of actions as the development of humans: that is, infinite development, if the next level is created from the standpoint of action with the body of man. If a machine acts together with a person, then it cannot run the person over, and therefore there is a single line of action — they are acting concurrently for the purpose of control.

And here is an important link: in order to determine in what way man sort of extricates himself from extreme situations, it is necessary to see that the goal of control in action of the One God in the physical body and man in the physical body — this goal is one. And so for each individual this goal is completely one. For example, if we look at the system which occurs in the course of advanced life support, then frequently the most important thing here is to identify the link connecting the person to the level of action together with God, that is, to remind him where he is acting together with God. And then, as it seems in extreme situations, when advanced life support measures are administered, at different levels of complexity of the systems, with complicated conditions — the person may recover, come out of a critical state, because he will have synchronized even in the past, that is, an element of the past in this case worked for him, as a level of action in the normal plane. So the way it works is that any action in the past can have a very practical significance, which can save a person. Therefore, any background history is providing redundancy and general improvement. In actual fact, it is creating a more powerful factor for subsequent development.

And from this viewpoint, for example, aging or depletion of the resources of the body — this looks somewhat like an abstract system. The question is only why it is being implemented. So, if we start from the standpoint of the One God, who has a physical body in one place, then, if we see that a crack appeared in the monolith stone, and this crack, from the standpoint of the One God, is action, which is defined as action of physical matter. The One God has physical matter, for example, in the form of a human body. And the stone has cracked, so that means that some element of destruction is happening here, which has a sign, generally speaking, of very generic development. That is, if the stone has cracked, this is clear throughout all the information as a crack, and therefore, it is possible to transfer information onto the physical body; it is sort of not necessary to touch any specific organ, but, it is possible that it affects the body's resources. That is, the stone was strong, and suddenly it cracked; that is, some event occurred, which tells us that there is some critical value. So if in the World some purely natural catastrophes exist, that affects the genetic composition of humans. And so to synchronize with the external part of nature this level is introduced: the level of genetic response; that is the level of aging due to the fact that there are some elements that are destructible, the elements of information transformation. But it is very easy to overcome this system, simply by developing knowledge to such a level that it is not necessary to react to the cracked stone. And by the way, the system of rejuvenation or regeneration works in a very powerful way: when any nearby object is detected, for example that same stone or torn leaf, and it is simply blocked out.

That is, how is it possible at all for a person to be rejuvenated? He just has to set up a screen to block out — not the people, but the external elements, which affect the genetic components, they implement the mechanism of the uniqueness of the system. If the stone cracked, the leaf fell — this is a quality which is unique and uniform, and it applies to humans as well. Each element of reality has equal conditions and equal elements of penetration into all areas of information. And so if this thread is sort of removed, then it is possible to calmly rejuvenate or recover, if the element of disease is related to some element of this type.

Actually, in my practice there was a case when I regenerated a renal duct. Then there was regeneration of a segment of the pancreas — not a very large area, about two centimeters, which physically did not exist. And I used the same universal case — the case of blocking out the falling leaf, just that; in information when this is introduced you can see it. So one and the same type of action results in the same changes of external, as it might seem, reality.

Or, what is the viral nature of some diseases? They spread as an element which is adequate to the external attributes of the environment. That is, if you capture a virus in an open location where it moves, and impose it, as if through a large magnifying glass, onto the environment, it is possible to identify a form which corresponds to the external environment, even though the environment may vary. Therefore, the virus sort of emulates the environment and destroys the organism — the discrete system of the environment, of course. And therefore, what should be done to get rid of the virus? Let us consider, for example, the case of atypical pneumonia, which exists in the World at this time. Here the virus, for example, has an ability to spread rapidly which is identical to that of smallpox, that is, viral in nature; if we were to plot a function, even though it would look slowed down to a considerable extent, but in this case we would see, among others, a cholera element added. That is, the way it works is that the virus develops in the general phase of information as a system, which simply restructures the body. And taking into account that the effort to quickly develop a vaccine at the mechanical, anti-material level has not been successful, it starts to change. If the original form is smallpox, which, however, works differently — in general. That is, there is the action of smallpox, and then there is, so to speak, a substrate of the virus itself; then the counteraction to this disease is, in view of this technology, a very simple one. All you have to do is to take a look, and project the virus — that is, to see to which element of the external environment it is attached, because this pertains to any viral series; having seen the discrete correspondence, it is simple to break the chain: create the action, which originates from a human who conforms with the norm.

Therefore, the next law of action with the one body of man is normalizing the situation. At every level of action there is normalization in the direction in which that physical body of man should also develop eternally and have the same level of subsequent development, as the body of God — that is, in the ideal case. Of course, God provides demonstration and teaches people, and as soon as people attain that as well, God acquires a different level of the body, the level of universality etc. The matter in question is that the local physical body would not be destroyed. And then, as it happens, we have a technology of counteraction, for example, of wars, technology guaranteeing 100%, that we will not end up with the destruction of everybody; simply because action together with the physical body of God shows us — a very simple option — as one human regards another.

God, which is in the future — He is indestructible, because He created; He will not allow self-destruction. The mechanism of creation does not contain the mechanism of destruction, in actual fact. That is, why will God not destroy himself? If you ask the question just so. The reason is, because the mechanism created originally, taking into account all the connections at once — it does not contain a mechanism for destruction. That was God's original idea, and so He created it. And therefore, the initial idea, that is, the construction, that is, the plan — exists in the consciousness of God. The consciousness of God, then, exists prior to his action. He first contemplates and then acts. But in the consciousness we perceive that as a consecutive value — what I have started with now; that is what the man is trying to attain when he wants to see the body of God. And having seen it, he immediately obtains all the information concerning the norm. Just by seeing it, even in his thought, by properly seeing the right points, let alone by seeing it physically.

By the way, that is why many Saints are such that it is impossible to approach them, the light bars the way, the light from the Creator, from the One God. And just seeing that light it seems to affect vision — in a physical way too. But during this there is powerful regeneration; the regenerative effect is very serious in the sense that the regeneration itself, it is, in general, rather prolonged; that is, the person at the same time falls into the field of the norm of the events, approaching the Saint. And this level, in general, which exists simply for the Saint, who is enlightened due to technology or some experience in reincarnation. And here, when we talk about the body of the One God, then here concurrently two values exist, as attributes of the full light — that is, the light, which does not let someone pass through, but at the same time there is even greater simplicity of access to this God. Because the issue of access, in essence, is just the question of the fact that God gives a greater possibility to approach Him, then to a Saint who is in the light of this light wave, as it happens, God should be more accessible. He should be seen at once by all people and accessible. Therefore, if a Saint so desires, he can also allow anyone to approach; and for this he needs to come out of the shining phase. The question is, then, to what extend does a Saint need that?

So the person doing the controlling, seeking to save everyone, must be able to work with any phase — of the highest shining or direct access, where it is needed. For example, during the treatment of malignant processes it is better to have the shining phase sometimes. If, however, dealing with a different type of disease — for example, the musculoskeletal systems, bones — then it is the other way round: it is necessary to work at the background level. That is, therefore, the same way as in healing: the action, the direction of action and regulation of one's own level are selected depending on the goal. And if we have, for example, the level of control, which relates to the fact that we receive control, in fact, as a goal — that is, control is exerted when the specific goal is known — then, that given goal exists in the events, and at the same time it is provided by God; then, we must understand Him in action, in reaching the goal. Therefore, we are always approaching God, including God in the physical body. Therefore, any action is the process of approaching, if it is a constructive action. Why it is constructive, that is, for example, salvation of all and action with respect to control through this using its own systems, private tasks — is the principle of creativity, which sort of goes from the general to the specific.

But if we consider, for example, why the non-destructive option allows us to approach closer, among other aspects. Because initially God was created in the process of construction and creation. It is impossible to create using the technology of destruction, and therefore the approach is constructive creation, and constructive creation means approaching the one body of God. Therefore when we come to this logically then your personal control now should be as follows: you should, as simply as that, create the following construct for control. Let's take, for example, personal tasks, and sort of locate them at the level where, when the physical body of God is acting in implementation of the issues; then it is as if you are talking [to Him] as a person, simply with another [person], who has a physical body. And in view of that the conversation may be taking into consideration the spiritual aspects, that is, spiritual expression; and so, having set forth the purpose of control in spiritual expression in the dialogue with the physical body of God, it means that you receive control of the kind which frequently happens between individuals — when this conversation sort of warms you, the implementation of the event is in progress, etc. And here all you have to do is simply come to the physical body of God, and it should be done unambiguously. It should not be in your imagination, but specifically, that you in fact enter in spiritual contact with God. But when you come into spiritual contact with God, then here you see that the Spirit of God is an expression of His physical body; and it makes it simpler for you. And therefore, you can decide, by doing something as simple as entering this state, that God has a physical body; you bring up your problem in front of yourself, and it is resolved, because this is the way you see reality.

And now you are performing this exercise; in fact it is not even an exercise — it is specific practice. What you should do: bring up your tasks in front of yourself; the One God, he is specifically in front of you, that is, he is in front of each one: so that it is possible to interact mentally and even physically. And most importantly, it must be the one and only physical body of the One God. When you come out and you resolve the issues even though in invisible mode, that is, it is resolved, because you are in spiritual contact, coming from the Spirit of God; moreover, from the Spirit of God, who has a physical body; not just a God in the generic understanding but specifically the physical body.

And so you will see how quickly the issues can be resolved. Here the issues are resolved practically at once, organically, as if no problem had ever existed. So, come out into this range, come out and affix yourself in this specifically.

Now you will do some work, and I will be working together with you...

For example, if this issue were to be considered: if we see specifically the body of God at the physical level, why does it become simpler to resolve issues pertaining to the spiritual plane, that is, in principle — logical or social issues, or issues of health, but at the spiritual plane? Because, in essence, when we are speaking about the way God is manifested, for example, in nutrition, how is his action manifested? Since nutrition is the ability of the human physical body to regenerate, maintain its functionality for the future. And so it goes, that when a person is eating, then at the same time — well, it depends on what products there are — for example, if he is eating bread it means he is approaching the understanding of cooperation with the physical body of God, and it can reach the level of the absolute.

Here another issue is the level of products which have some functional or applied purpose. Therefore here we are looking at the situation where — if we consider drinking — the concept of „drink“ may be such a concept, that you could drink, for example, wine, or water, but it is liquid. So the characteristics of liquid are uniform and generic, that is, they are universal from the standpoint of the One God. Therefore wine may have the same characteristics as water, for example, or the other way round. That is, for the One God this is, generally speaking, the same product. Here is His perception of liquid: He created water, and then He also created grapes, from which wine is made, that is, at the level of the Spirit it is the same product. And when you work with the physical body of the One God you obtain the universal system of control, which has a multifactor meaning. Because here you receive, in essence, the same level of reactivity, which comes from the level, in essence, of the organization of your

Soul, the original level. Because for the Soul, at the point of its original organization, all the phenomena are practically identical as at the original point, at the instance, when God self-organized. And so it happens, that implementation of the level of the Soul in spiritual action is connected to simply the interaction between the physical bodies of the One God and the human which He created.

Therefore, based on that, it is possible to conclude that joint actions of people created in the image — are also actions of the Soul. That is, the Soul knows precisely why this person is in this place and why he is supposed to do something specifically here, even though from the standpoint of logic and consciousness the person may still be asking questions — why is it so. And therefore I believe that here is a lot to learn from the simple level of contact of people, interactions of people. And in this case here one just needs to input the level, in essence of the presence of the One God, where it will be clear, why at this time the situation is the way it is. Because for God, who has created people — all people — it is completely clear why things are that way. When you create a certain construct, it is clear to you why you placed one level or another in a certain way and location. And based on this analogy we can say that we can determine precisely the object of the action, or any element of reality for that matter, if we simply follow this logical conclusion described below: if it is clear for God why people have gathered or some events are occurring, then if you are the one performing the action it is clear to you as well.

But if you comprehend it using the Spirit, then you might be able to see a different reality, a remote one that pertains to spiritual vision or clairvoyance, that depends on what you use for understanding. And so it goes that the understanding Spirit, that is, the Spirit that is acquiring knowledge is the level which corresponds to the fact that the Spirit striving for knowledge is always a multifactor entity. That is, it can unite everyone and everything as a sublevel, the way the One God does, or it can, in practice, sort of see the individual picture, preserving the individuality and yet at the same time remaining the unifying factor for all. And that's why. When we are talking specifically about the Spirit, for example, about the Holy Spirit, that is, the external Spirit coming from the body of God, then we see that the level of unification in this case is brought down to the fact that we visualize the picture of action of the Spirit of God, that is, acting practically, traveling towards the body of man, as if from the One God, and at the same time coming from the Spirit of man itself: the self-restoring Spirit, the Spirit that organizes the body.

And so when the spiritual impetus organizes the body, then any environment — or absolutely any system — will be conducive to the body being normal and organized. And so these so called discrete systems which I have mentioned with respect to situations involving viruses — they become ineffective if the Spirit is at the level of their understanding. That is, in this case the virus becomes non-functional. And generally speaking, any disease will become non-functional — that is it will then be cured. If spiritual characteristics are such that you will be able to, in the state of the Spirit and in the state of the physical body, introduce both the parameter of individuality and the parameter of universality. Because, if there is the external level, the parameter of universality, and you introduce it as the controlling system, for example, over some processes, then as soon as you bring it into an organism as an action this system will take control and be controlled by you. That is, you can control the system, because the signal is located inside of you.

So, for what purpose were the senses of humans created? If you ask yourself this simple question. So, man has senses, functional action for what purpose? How do you work using feelings and senses together with action using the physical body of man? We are talking, so far, about a somewhat undefined area of action, for example, action together with the body: when you wave your hand, and obtain a complete cure, and reach the event level, all the concurrent spiritual actions.. If we are talking about the level of action with the physical body of God, then here it is possible to consider the following issue. Because for God the feelings of man and his physical body are basically systems of the same level, again, from the universal standpoint of God. Then, if we, for example, have the level of control that we want to understand what to do with respect to acting using the senses together with the physical body of God, then it should be clear to us that the external action is such that when you are controlling a certain event, then you are not considering, within this event what elements are occurring, and where, and you control them somewhere using spiritual content.

So here it is possible to see what to do with the feelings together with the physical body of God, if you introduce an external control of sorts — the control of will, or visual, etc. So it goes, that if we have a level of control aimed at some specific action, then here the level of objectification of action, that is, the external control in this case — is, in fact, your physical body, that is, the sign of the objective character of action for God and for you is your physical body. And taking into account that sign of objectification, as a certain pillar of reality, it should generally be eternal. That is, the goal of God is such that the factor of objectification, that is, the factor of convergence, or factor, somewhat to a greater extent, of simultaneity of action, this physical body, which is supposed to be eternal. Because God acts with respect to an eternal task, and He must certainly act in accordance with the levels, which are eternal, sort of fix those levels with the eternal constructs, in fact. The body, following this principle, is supposed to be eternal. And when you understand this principle, then you see: it is sufficient to introduce the parameter of external control, to consider the principle of eternal existence of the body due to the task of action of God, and then it will be clear that feelings acting together with the physical body of God — this is the parameter of revealed external reality. That is — and you have to pay attention now — frequently feelings sort of open the World for you, it's some sort of door; and this, by the way, is an extremely powerful regenerative mechanism of the human organism. If you open it up correctly, here you are — healthy. Also, frequently the organism can be completely restored by just a single fleeting feeling by association: sort of an instantaneous system of regeneration. That is, the person falls into his own pillar, the matrix pillar that is, and since he was restored, that means that he had walked in a place where God had specified a task for him. Well, maybe he did not walk there physically, but he walked along the right path.

And therefore I am bringing in this concept: the concept of attaining actions. There is a concept of karmic systems, in order to save a nuclear power plant or a planet from global destruction; this may frequently burden the cause and effect systems. And in order to attain a result, it is necessary to simply enter a system, like a plug, and introduce the parameters there and immediately everything will be saved. That is, this so-called plug is some system of the norm; it is somewhere where the actions of God and the cumulative effect of man in terms of feelings, actions, and in the physical body are all aligned.

I have already introduced the next level, when not only feelings, revealing the World, create the World — that is, as it happens, an element of the creation of the World from the human side is the plane of feelings, and the first and foremost one is the Love of man. And when man loves the World, he can build, in principle, any element of reality, and generally move various objects, materialize things, etc. This is a sort of manifestation of Love. Love in this understanding produces the norm. That is, another person does not suffer from it: just the opposite, he gains development. And when you receive a premeditated action — why would you move anything, for example; if it is needed for salvation to a great extent, it is possible to materialize a major element, say, a plane in flight, for some purpose. But it is possible to set an objective: to place a small grain on the table and sit over it for a long time; but if it is not included in the task of concurrent action and purpose of the One God in all His manifestations, including the physical body (already, the other way round, in this case God is manifested everywhere), then it can become a very lengthy task, before things are synchronized and this grain of sand is materialized.

That is, the objective of the action is determined, first and foremost, by the proportionality of mindfulness. It is understandable when people are walking together, they reasonably accommodate to give others space on the sidewalk, and there is a level of sort of logical reasonability of action. So, the level of logical reason of action in these processes is universal salvation. So, that already everything is so clear that everyone must be redeemed and live eternally; and originally logically this is clear as well, and even proceeding from the practice of the development of civilization, that when we see the elements of the plane of destruction as elements proceeding into a certain reality, it is possible to regard them as elements which are very old that have appeared prior to the element of the primary action: of the One God.

That is, any type of destruction, for example, war is an element „preceding the action". Because action is always creation and construction. So then the question arises: what is the concept „preceding the action of God"? God created everything, carried out one single action — and the World appeared. So in this case „preceding the action of God" — is a factor, where the single body of God is manifested, either as bringing universal salvation, the light or in the way, that the single body of God does not allow the appearance of certain factors. Supposing, since He is indestructible, naturally, He can appear in areas where military action is in progress. But since He is universal and that covers everybody, so if a person may be affected by military action, He will not come there. He does not stop the military action, for example, by the move of His hand. Because where there is development there is civilization, first of all.

But the true principle „preceding the action of God“ — it is the principle of a sort of undefined system. That is, if the system is defined, for example, there is positive action — it is defined as strongly positive, and the system starts developing, then „preceding the action of God“ is something that does not designate this system. That is, a certain look at the level of equality and complete freedom that the system of creative construction must develop into a defined system. From the standpoint of any element of reality, if we want to understand what the undefined systems are, and take any element of reality there: air, vacuum — it perceives a developing, positively developing World as a system which may still be undefined for its level of reality.

For example, a speck of dust; what difference does the development of civilization make for a speck of dust? But in fact it makes a big difference. Everything is a sign of collective consciousness. And this very speck of dust is located at this point and no other as a sign of some material substrate of the World generally. And so if the development goes this way, then so it goes — any actions of a seemingly antagonistic nature in the plane of constructive creation — this indicates that the developing World, in fact, does not define the precise trajectory of development. That is, for example, there is a car moving; it can move through some kind of thicket, bumping against the trees; or it can come out onto a road and move normally. So, when we develop a World, the level „preceding the action of God“ — well, let's put it this way — as to why negative information exists — this is really simply just a level of this type; that what God provides, what can be done in general, but we just simply are not using that. We are driving down the road there, just so, and this car may be bumping up against trees. That is, the overall question is that of personal freedom.

Because God created man in His image, which includes, inter alia, the physical body of man. Therefore he must choose: either he drives and has the knowledge, that is, receives the knowledge and develops properly, or he does not want to. Therefore, this level „preceding the action of God" — this is no more than an element of personal choice, which is so perceived by man. That is, man may perceive that God did not here exert an action originally. And therefore all the wars and all that— this is very old information, which existed before the first signs of creative action. I, generally speaking, put in the data and modeled the control in this manner, because in this way it was convenient to record the negative level of information using the marker that it was older, darker, and possessed characteristics pertaining to an earlier point, before the signs of the constructive action.

When we take over this control, and by the way, this is the way it is in reality — when we take over this control and receive the result that we know these characteristics, we see that characteristics start dissolving all by themselves. That is, the principle of discovery is the principle of action. That is, if we know what comes from where then we can resolve the issue very simply. Therefore, any problem can be resolved by identifying in it simply the earliest attribute from the standpoint of so to speak negative range, and simply by adding, compressing the time to a more modern point, that is, by increasing the speed of time on the negative level.

From the standpoint of Divine action this is very logical. In an infinite amount of time everything will become normal anyway. And we sort of set the time counter to a faster rate — and receive the norm. By the way, during resuscitation, in measures taken to ensure rapid regeneration or emergency response, people frequently feel that everything slows down, according to their perception. So, this slowing down — this means that the Soul is growing towards the World. Soul sort of bends the World to fit it and partially overtakes control of this, already acting to a greater extent together with the physical body of indestructible God. Then as a result the person does not perish, etc.

Here sometimes it is manifested in people as an element of control, because at that moment the person understands how the physical body of God is set up, how it functions, and how it interacts. Because for God, actually, there is no difference whether it is body, or air; to Him all is one. He created the air, that is, for him these are objects of the same order of magnitude, and so control from this standpoint is perfect — extremely simple, in general.

If we have, for example, this picture, then it would seem that if it is the same environment, so then there is a sign of differentiation, so that's why God created people so diverse, following different goals of their own. So if you look at His tasks, the diverse environment is a sign of objectivization of action from the standpoint of the fact that God Himself creates a structure in a particular way because He needs it. That is, „objectivization" and „needs" from the standpoint of His freedom of will. That is, any manifestation of the World is also the compete freedom of will of action of the One God. And so it goes then, that we have an interconnection as to why a human needs freedom, because God is acting in a way which is being absolutely free. And an option of co-action, an option of concurrent action — this is, again, the absolute freedom of man. He created in His image, so He cannot restrain [man] in anything at all. And so here appears the following element: in order to obtain the universal from action together with the physical body if God, it is necessary to act as if together with the physical body — this is clear, but it is possible to act, unlike the way they do in common systems, using feelings in exactly the same way as action with the physical body.

Pay attention — I am introducing this system of control in general for the first time, because namely the volitional action by the sensual plane equals the action of the physical body, in case of contact with the one body, specifically physical body of the One God. This is the first time I am introducing this construct, therefore here you have to pay extra attention today: it is being shown for the first time, because here very strong controlling points appear, and of what type are they? Any movement of the physical body may lead to control, but it is possible to use the plane of feelings to affect physical reality. Therefore, this is an identical level of control. That is, the feelings plane — it includes both the parameters of the senses and the plane of instant access. When we perceive using the senses or feelings, we frequently do not perceive that here it is somewhere in some local place. This is the universal level of access, and therefore the work proceeding here is universal. And here you just have to pay extra attention, because feeling must be correlated with your physical body, that is, it should sort of come forth from the level of the physical body, sort of from inside, from the heart. That is, you must clearly understand that feeling comes forth from you — this is the first criterion. And the second criterion — this is that you must, having at least once seen the one body of God, that is, the physical body of God, even if using remote vision, fixate yourself; best of all if you do it at the spiritual level of interconnection.

That is the advantage: when you tune in to the physical body of the One God, frequently you do not need to go high up into the informational access level. Supposing, God forbid, that there is some extreme critical situation, for example, it is neccesary to make an urgent decision regarding an aircraft, which has some problem. If you go to the level of technology and access it on the spiritual plane — it's simply too long, and meanwhile time is passing. But if you remember God as a human, that provides instant control. Therefore in extreme systems, by tuning in to the physical body of God, you receive practically instantaneous control, and in addition, it happens immediately. But this is not necessarily used only for instantaneous systems of control, it can be used and control may be applied, of course, for resolving any tasks. Moreover, here the spiritual level is what provides this practical stability in action. Therefore when here you receive control, in fact total control, for basically a one-time action, then the sign of universal salvation here, according to my teaching „On Salvation and Harmonious Development“ is the fact that the One God is alive, He is here nearby, therefore, naturally everyone is saved. He is the guarantor of salvation for everyone.

This completes our workshop today. If possible, practice intensively, at the same time obtaining knowledge from the state which occurs during interaction with the body of the One God with the physical body.

Thank you for your attention.

Method of Approaching the Physical Body of the One God

April 21, 2003

Good afternoon.

The topic of today's seminar is the implementation and dissemination of my „Teaching on Salvation and Harmonious Development", and the subtopic is — „Method for Approaching the Physical Body of the One God „. This method can be viewed as approaching the common physical body of the One God, that is, the specifically physical approach, the spiritual approach, using the Spirit, etc. Similarly [it] can be viewed as follows: when the One God created the physical body of man, then here the question specifically is what the physical body should be — this question is unequivocally resolved in the direction that the body in this case is physically ideal from the standpoint of the One God. Therefore since He created the ideal physical body, then even approaching his physical body means understanding the canons of the ideal physical body, that is, the good — which means normal — physical condition, good to the maximum extent, and interaction with the Spirit, Soul and consciousness, etc.

In view of that, when we are talking about movement towards the one physical body of the One God, specifically to His single body, in this case the term „one" implies that God has his own specific single physical body, and here we can see, first and foremost, the procedure of organization of the physical body by the One God Himself. That is, in what way the One God created his own physical body. And then we come to the solution of this question as being the question with which we have become familiar from the standpoint of human practice, because God, who created man, naturally in a way projected what He had created for Himself onto humans.

Therefore it is immediately clear: in order for the body to be felt by the Spirit, if we state that the Spirit is the external creating substance, so for the body to become self-aware and develop itself, for this some differentiations in self-perception are needed. For example, a person is walking: it means that there should be ground since he has to walk on something; there should be air, etc. And so there is this flow of the external, flow of what moves faster than the speed of movement of the images; for example, the person steps on the ground, walks along a path somewhere, and some physical objects are coming towards him. So the objects are also there because of the Creator, the One God; they have been created in the same manner before they are perceived as images. For the One God any object of information exists specifically in this moment, that is, it is created precisely at this moment, and for it there is no concept of „past“, „future“, etc.; there is the specific concept „now“, in this case, now, from the creation at this time. Which, of course, has the future, and had the past in relation to this event.

So, if we were to consider this issue as follows: let's take as a comparison, for example, a truck, where there is a driver, and which has a cabin and a number of trailers. And so if those trailers to the truck we were to consider as a sequential element: that is, first the truck starts moving and then the trailer, and if a person is just watching the trailer from the side and sees a moving trailer, logically he understands that it must be pulled by the truck. Because he generally understands the design of the trailer: it is unable to move by itself; in a rare case it may move down a slope if someone pushes it first. So here in addition the person has this sign of recognition related to the movement of the sequential part; this exists from God, from the One God, practically a priori, that is, it has existed from the beginning. And in view of that so it goes that this particular sign of recognition, which exists in the way of so called logical knowledge of the truck — for the person it has been set forth from the body of the One God.

So here I have explained that when a person learns of the elements of physical reality he perceived them precisely as the elements of physical reality, sort of causality, as a „trailer“, of sorts, to something original. So by analogy with the movement of the truck, where the cabin works as a source, in fact, here the specific element of the body of man serves as the element of recognition. So this specific element of the body of man is physical human blood. That is, the element of blood is the element of recognition. But in principle, the way blood works is that it moves throughout the organism, and all the time recognizes the next element of reality. Because it moves itself, for a number of specific reasons — for example, the heart is working, etc., but also because those functions are embedded in the blood. That is, from the standpoint of the One God the function itself contains the external form.

Because for God from the standpoint of the design of the physical body of the One God, that form and that movement of the blood is basically the same thing. One is sort of contained within the other. And if we look at the issue, for example, of why the blood does not flow out of the body, why it does not ooze out of the capillaries? Understandably, there are some dense tissues. But in the overall scheme of things if we consider specifically the physical body of the One God, there the blood does not flow out of the body because this blood, after all, has been projected in the form of the specific events of the external World, and it does not have anywhere to flow out to. For the One God external events are the same as internal ones. And that's why back in his time Jesus also said that it is blood — when they drink wine, and he compared it with blood. Right? He compared them in a more precise position — here the wine specifically is regarded, for example, as the blood of Jesus. Therefore, in terms of external reality that object is comparable with the internal content, for example, of Jesus. Here we can see that this comparison is a specific act in order to improve the health, for example, of the blood of any person as an organizing substance: it is sufficient to equalize the external object of reality. That is, to make it so that the external environment into which blood could flow out or somehow be changed, for example in the case of a possible adverse scenario — those elements just need to be brought under control to the norm.

Then the question arises, what elements are those? We are talking already not only about healing, but about control in general at any level of event. So in accordance with my „Teaching On Salvation And Harmonious Development", dissemination of information pertaining to any one signal, one element — for example, healing — this is, in essence, still universal information, that is, this technology is suitable for any level, including the level of salvation of all. So in order to not have the element of possible leakage it is necessary again to bring in the system of salvation of all. Then as it happens, He will save himself in that moment. So that's why the self-enclosed, as it seems, target objective — to save all — in fact it is the task for the solution at the same time, that is, that way lies the solution of the issue, of the task itself.

So the term „task of the solution" — it is a special term, and one has to pay attention here. And when we have control here, the way it works is that it is control of the so called remote type, that is, any element of reality — the segments closest to you in consciousness, in Spirit. That is, the organizing Spirit is located right next to you, you can affix the point of your organizing Spirit. The Spirit which organizes reality. Because there is the learning Spirit, the joyful Spirit, etc. And your Spirit which organizes reality is what is the closest to you, to your physical body. When it is very close, the Spirit matches the body. And against the background of this matching you will see how your heart is being created by the Spirit. During this it is created not in the form of a physical organ, but in the form of a causal system — the movement of blood. That is, the Spirit immediately creates a stable future process, and so it goes that you have a stable future because the Spirit is working, which initially creates the body itself.

So the principle of self-creation here is that He will not create in reality some kind of hole into which blood would flow, for example, and change. Therefore, you can drink any quantity of wine, but the blood from Jesus will not at all diminish, and therefore; as it happens that this is eternal life, because everything, that is reproduced from the outside, that is, what is drunk, or eaten, does not in any way affect the internal system of the physical body of the One God. And here we can see that if something, for example, is eaten as His body, the body may be (God is manifested in animals, etc.) in the form, for example, of actions of a particular animal or a particular element of reality. But in accordance with the Divine task in the future, any object has to be initially equalized, that is, as an intellectual level, the level, for example, of events; for any object of information these levels must, generally speaking, be equalized. If the person has the level of complete freedom, then in the future an animal should attain a level of a certain personal freedom, that is, it should not be sort of eaten in accordance with ongoing biological processes. And here the issue, to a greater extent, is that sort of the matrix system is eaten, what reproduces this animal. It is the level of the horn of plenty. There it is possible to keep eating everything all the time, and the horn, it sort of always stays inexhaustible. Well, not sort of, actually — it does, in fact, stay inexhaustible.

And so here an element appears, that when you are working towards reality from the standpoint of the specifically physical body of the One God, that is, to create reality, you are creating it — the appearing element autonomously in a closed system, that is, you are creating it on your own. Therefore, you must have all the resources coming from you, that is, the World must infinitely develop from you, and you will stay inexhaustible during this process. This is the principle. And so then, if we, for example, are considering the level of this, let's put it this way, plane of identical development of everybody, and everyone should in the end be equal, with equal rights. Let us assume, in the constitution of the state of Grigori there is that point defined at which the equality of all objects of information is a state, including the animal kingdom, etc. And in view of that, here the element of control is also embedded in the fact that equality is the reverse position, which we create ourselves, but the position specifically of the One God, because as God, He is generally equal to everybody from the start.

It is just that man, specifically in terms of freedom of choice somehow or other changes the structure of events: either following the line coming from the One God, or he, for example, in some way comes out and starts the restoration process later. So when we are talking, for example, about cancerous processes, then in this case, if we look, for the sake of an example, at the human organism and state, that there is a tumor in this case. So the tumor is, inter alia, from the standpoint of this position, a situation in which the external picture of physical reality becomes unbalanced, and the external World sort of pushes through at one of the points, not necessarily at the point of the tumor, and somewhere the structure is replaced, that is, as a foreign body. It is clear that it must have come from somewhere.

And in view of that, for normalization — not only for cancerous processes, but for normalization of the situation in general in which there is external influence, the element of control is deep internal self-organization. That is, initially from the purity of the one physical body of God, where a tumor cannot even consider appearing — there everything is sufficiently equalized; everything is very compensated. Therefore when a person sort of comes to the internal pure source within himself, then it is so, that we have in this source the system of absolutely complete self-regeneration, and an instantaneous one at that. And then it is completely unclear why the tumor frequently disappears without a trace — such a large growth, and all of a sudden it is gone, for example. Or there is an event which has the strongest external influence, and suddenly the external source disappears, and it is as if there were no problems at all, and never were, most importantly. So here the element is equalization of the World in this method of control from the standpoint of the one physical God, manifested in the physical body, that is, specifically in a body of man, in a physical human body.

When we are considering this statement at an axiomatic level — the words that were said, for example, „one physical body of God", then here appearing as a human at the human level, are in a deeper structure, in the next structure. Because from the standpoint of logic, in order for the person, for example, to move about, he should be able to step on something, there should be ground. So it goes that initially the physical body of God, through development of one's own, consciousness results; through logic the element is brought forth out of a deeper attitude towards oneself, to one's own physical body of the One God. And it is precisely the deeper attitude to oneself that brings forth physical reality, actually. That is, this element of bringing forth physical reality — it's actually there sort of from the start. This is the process that is embedded in man as a process of recognition, for example, of another person from any distance.

If, let us suppose, there is a question as to whether there is life anywhere besides, for example, planet Earth, then recognition is the element most closely present in man. If it is necessary to diagnose some galaxy or universe to see if there is life, for example, then the closest area, the wave level, when the external World forces another person more, not in any negative way, but just at a diagnostic level, as a system of diagnostics, that is the presence of something living — in any form.

There was a time when I provided a prediction with respect to vegetation on Mars, and later a satellite actually discovered chlorophyll — discovered it at that very location. That is, even though I published this prediction, there is the action of collective consciousness in it with respect to work on that aspect — which contributes to the fulfillment of the prediction. But later, it is true, a satellite already went by there, but still there is a controlling action. It is possible, for example, to exert control, and why should we not materialize those, for example, chlorophyll molecules, and not create this vegetation remotely, it might seem. But on the other hand, this, generally speaking, is actually possible, I am convinced. But as a practice — it should be possible to confirm. But when we check for confirmation it all depends on what method we use. If we are checking using a satellite as a method, then, well, it could be true, in fact chlorophyll could be present there, but there could be not just chlorophyll. There can be a situation there such that chlorophyll itself is not, strictly speaking, the causal level. The matter there could pertain more to such systems, such as that water is present there, and, on the basis of that water, chlorophyll reproduces in some vegetative systems like ferns. Therefore here we have, strictly speaking, not just chlorophyll itself, but again we have a more coherent system; it is deeper, it seems, just with the diagnostics: if we just bring up the issue concerning vegetation, we again end up with a deeper system, in that connection. So here as well we can say that the external system of observation determines some status of the event. Supposing, chlorophyll on Mars or vegetation on Mars — it is water, the fern in the end consists of chlorophyll, etc. Then we have these specific features here: first of all, before, prior to the flight of this satellite, for the first time, by the way, and it was determined not so long ago, that chlorophyll, that some green vegetation was present, and that it was green. It was believed before that there was no proof. That is, in principle, even though they talked a lot, however, I provided the information that was mine, that is, I mobilized, of course, the collective consciousness of the people.

For example, there is a projection — life appeared, because, where control over life is exerted, that's where life appears, of course. But if the satellite previously did not go over that area very often, it is possible that it could not notice it. So here this system appears that the logical phase of control, specifically what is related to the logic of the process, this level is sort of very closely connected to the viewpoint. So, if on Mars there were, for example, some permanently stationed astronaut, and chlorophyll appeared in front of him, we would say, yes, now we have launched into the picture of consciousness this information; we would say — this is a clean experiment. But since here, first of all, it is technically far — very far — that is, we cannot do it instantly; there is no astronaut there, on the surface of Mars; so therefore we are using the access of the spiritual plane, sort of, which takes into account the multiple dimensions of possible actions.

So, this system of multiple angles in information — this is the system of control, which can build physical reality, practically before the physical body of the One God. But with this to build it in the way as indefinite systems are specially created. Because the One God, He creates everything, including the undefined system, that is, picking through options is a created system. And when we perceive the searching through options, then considering, for example, the position with respect to resurrecting people, we see that no options are available there at all. A person, if he is born, is a single entity — a level without options; therefore where no options are available — the system there, in fact, is originally infinite. If we consider — then why should the plants be so close with respect to the level of independence, freedom of man: then they will also fall in the same status and have a different type of development. That is, it will be possible to eat a plant, but without consuming it. So this is the approximate type.

That is, there is no such level where the World is altered with respect to the one physical body of the One God. Because where control is diminished — it means there is a change there. And so the best level of restoration, including for the physical body, but in addition to the physical body also for the Soul, Spirit, and consciousness — is the level, when the person tries to minimally affect the external World. For example, like the Buddhist philosophy — not destroying anything.. But in this if, for example, we are talking already about the element of resurrection as a practical element, then it happens here that the method of resurrection, generally, is something that is simply understood.

So, the physical World, it is originally set up in such a way that where there are no options — this is already an original eternal environment, which, by analogy with the physical body of the One God, this environment, it is already immediately and automatically capable of organizing the next reality around itself, and generally, an infinite number of systems. If, for example, biological decay, physical death of man enters into this infinite reality then it means that it is no more than one of the options of multiplicity of variants. From the standpoint of the individual, the Soul of man, he can select another option — simply to rise back from the grave. But the most important thing is to know the technology and principle of the design and operation of this World.

And when we are talking about the cure as a system, for example, using the technology of resurrection, then it is the same level for complicated diseases, for example, of vascular systems, those which are the defining systems, generally speaking, of any systems; the element of control is to input future events into those systems which have become most weakened, input the macro-salvation. Those global systems: salvation from a possible explosion of a nuclear reactor, so that there is no global war. That is, generally speaking, in essence, this technology is very pragmatic, completely specific, strict, technologically a very clearly defined system of salvation — for the individual as well, even sometimes first and foremost for the individual.

For example, a person has some pathological systems in terms of health — it means that it is possible to restore it very quickly, if you insert the task of salvation specifically for all in the area of the weakest systems of events in the future. So then the way it works is that events of the future from the standpoint of man mean that he is strengtherning his path forward, that is, it is a permanent optimization system. Therefore the body, one body, the physical body of the One God, is what has, in the external system, what is most optimal for this physical body of the One God. That is, the , external environment for Him is, in fact, similar to a situation when somewhere along a street passes the One God in His physical body, and a human body, too, and He walks in that way because that external environment is at that level, the uniform option for him, because He covers all the versions of reality. And so then for a person to make a precise movement, he would still have to work with a certain number of options.

But when we work on the salvation of everyone, we arrive, accordingly, at a single option. However, if we set the objective of harmonious development, then we can bring the option as a logically conscious one, necessitated by past experience. Harmony is what a person always needs, let's put it that way. And therefore so it goes, that there is a necessary option, and then at the same time there is one that would suffice. If salvation of everyone is the necessary one, mandatory in case of problem-ridden systems of development, then the harmonious one is something that would generally suffice, but it is broader: it will suffice to ensure salvation even if there is universal harmony. What it comes to here is what is given from the One God, is sort of turning into an absolute, a reflexory mechanism set on top of what a person had done in terms of his consciousness, in terms of the next level of development, for example, harmony from the standpoint of the person.

So harmony from the standpoint of the person must coincide with harmony from the standpoint of the One God and in the same way, naturally, the physical body of the One God. The physical body of the One God is eternal. Therefore, for real harmony, the physical body of man must be eternal. So the, person must strive to ensure that the body develops and spreads; of course it is one entity on the plane of dissemination. That is, to put some effort into external reality, but the kind of effort that would lead to his body also developing in the same way as the physical body of the One God, the one physical body of God.

Then what we have here is a certain system of regularities related to the fact that control in this sense is the control of approaching the physical body of the One God. That is, as soon as a person approaches him — physically or spiritually — then he understands accordingly in what way in this instance the physical body of the One God operates. For example, what does He do?

When God is sitting in his sauna, does He use the birch sauna switches or not? And why at this particular moment is He not using them? So here sort of the analysis of correspondence shows us that doing it even without some special long-term systems of education, or with respect to direct action — it is always aimed at obtaining understanding, that is, we have a transfer of knowledge simply by the fact that the factor of the existence of the physical body of the One God transfers all the knowledge with respect to its internal design. Elementary for a person.

If a person runs out of the sauna and jumps into cold water, another person observing this may say: „Yes, so it's okay to do this if that one does not catch a cold „. He may not even know the basics of physiology at some kind of scientific level, but just jump. It is the same way if at some moment the One God in his physical body is not using switches in the sauna; so it means— He is doing it for some purpose. The first analogy is: a sauna switch is a bunch of branches that have been cut, right? So, for example, one should not cut, — this is the simplest version, etc. And here we come to the next level of laws and regularities — approximation through the external level provides the norm of events. And when you already approach further, analyzing the external systems of reality, you can see how the physical body of the One God was created: for example, having looked at reality in the round — because it is His manifestation. The norm of reality — this is how It was created.

If you take a large ball of thread and spread that thread in different directions, still, using the thread it is necessary to come to the reason for the ball — initially, where that ball was created. In the same manner the random network of physical events leads you. Since He is inseparably connected with the physical event, the quintessence of control here lies in the fact that when we approach the physical body of the One God we are following an unbreakable chain of events. And the physical World for us falls into the same level of perception as the informational World for a person when he, for example, is using a different system of control. And here both the physical and the informational World are all the same monolith, they are not distinguished in terms of movement, this is a special control system. It has a completely different level of stability, and in addition it has a different level from the standpoint of control movement — it is comprehensible. The purpose is very clear: simply to approach the physical body of the One God. And during the elements of acquiring knowledge you have to perform no more than elementary actions, try to understand if the One God in his physical body makes a movement of some kind — how to use this experience for yourself.

If we want, for example, if we need to look for edible berries in the forest, it is possible to use the technology of this. This is a specific technology, because berries are what spread from His physical body and are in an unbreakable bond with Him. So it goes, that this system of control — is a system, first, clear and understandable with respect to the goal, and secondly, it is performed naturally for the person. A person, while constantly doing something, is also doing other things at the same time. That is, this is most natural and it most harmoniously occurs from the standpoint of control systems common for a person.

And therefore — as a training exercise — now perform the following: take the goals which you have; place them in small spheres in front of yourselves and just perform control. So what is your goal of control, that is, your goal now, for example? And let these spheres develop in the direction of the physical body of the One God. Let them start to sort of unfurl and move in His direction, and you can see that any object of control is moving in the direction of Him towards the physical body of the One God. When you start seeing that, you see that the control is more intensive if these spheres are moving faster. This is like a control method. Now you work, and I will work together with you...

When the control is realized for you, you can see that the sphere has rolled up to the physical body of the One God, it is God who decides. In essence, any action is originally determined by God, the One God, the Creator, the Creator-God. Therefore so it goes that, as soon as you see, that the body of the One God touched your sphere — your issue has been resolved. Therefore, the criterion of correctness of movement is nothing more than simply the mechanical trajectory of movement of this sphere in the direction of the current location of the physical body of the One God.

And based on this, if we were to look how the development of the Spirit of the person is created by the person himself: he strives for actions personified from the actions of God or by God Himself, by some Divine actions, aimed at some kind of missions, some overriding system super-objectives. He does fulfill them though, for example, if there is a creative person. He sets them and fulfills them. The development coming from him by means of some tasks, affects physical reality: for example, Einstein's formula E= тс2, or an element in the form of fine arts, or generally speaking it may be any small invention

— like the wheel, for example — affects the external World, that is, it is an influence system.

How do you do it, if you set yourself this question — how to arrive at an invention that will certainly save everyone, just mechanically? I have now named an element which influences the physical World; so it is the simplest — the spiritual element, for example, as a method, as an invention. So it is, if we are talking about eternal development, then it is some system, which is changing. If we take, for example, the technology of eternal life of the physical body of a person. So then it means, that yes, if he knows, if one person knows — the whole system, and teaches everyone; and that means everyone will be saved. That is, for the overall development, we have, as a technology, that is, some developing system, which is not static in terms of logic so that it could have eternal development.

But if we have static development, then how do we transfer it into an eternal configuration for example, the same very wheel again. So it seems it is possible to transfer through a very large volume of actions related to the wheel in the development of the future. But in case of antigravity, the wheel does not seem to be needed. Again, there is a disconnect here. Or for an aircraft which lands on the water surface, the wheel may not be much needed. Already there are some exceptions. So then, the element of exception is the developing World, because when there were no planes, wheels were sufficient, in addition to, for example, horses, the horses' hooves. So here from the standpoint of contact with external moving reality, horses or carriages, or the soil, initially created by the One God, it looks as follows: subsequent development may sort of exclude the preceding level.

Then the concept of technology frequently contains a canonic element: faith. A believer, by the way, may be cured from a disease quickly: he simply is included in the system of true faith specifically, in the future norm of events, created by the One God. And then there are no problems: he will in fact be quickly and easily cured, that is, there are no problems at all, as a matter of principle. And how can a person acquire faith that is so reliable? So, he must somewhere meet, it looks like, and sort of make an agreement. He must, by analogy, meet with the physical body, simply with the One God in the physical body of a man: they meet, they agree, they shake hands and he acquires strong clear faith in this event. I am talking about that one element.

So, when this event is resolved, so they have agreed, so then does the person owe anything? The One God, He generally speaking, does not demand unconditional submission from the person. The person has to choose for himself. So, he says: „Yes, I will do this and that". That's all — it is agreed, the event is resolved. And therefore it means, that absolutization of the faith... why resurrect Jesus, for example, inasmuch as at a level of his eternal physical body this is the question, in general of absolute faith, sort of precision of the path. Yes, of course, there are other religious systems as well; I am just providing an example of a concession from one of those. So then we have the level of development, related to the comparable actions of the person; if a person agreed with another, shook hands or signed an agreement — he had seen his physical body.

Because he, the person, in principle — could make agreements with a tree, if he knows how to use telepathy. But what about the tree? It does not sign anything, for example. It is only possible to make agreements telepathically. So the difference between what is in action and what is static — what is it? With respect to the tree the person is the controlling system. And the tree, in principle, can only passively offer forth some products that it produces. And so it goes, that any controlling level implies that the level of its faith, sort of the guarantor of reliability, should be more of a controlling system or a comparable one. So, the comparable one is, again, the physical body of the One God. At that level He sort of enters into the specific systems of agreement.

And so, when we consider such a condition as sleep in humans, we shall see that this entrance of the external World into the person when the person is asleep (he frequently feels in sleep some actions which resemble the actions of the physical in the World or in the pre-physical World), then here this entrance in fact does occur, in fact, the entrance, that is, the passage, which practically goes from the physical body of the One God to the body of the person. But during this the passage is not performed in an obvious way; that is, the One God must approach everyone: He is not going to multiply when He has one physical body, the same as a person. He, if we look at it from the other side, is created in the same way a person is, if you look from a person's side. And therefore he can enter through some mechanism, which is at the same time the same for everyone, oh well, maybe at different times, for example, through sleep. And so that entrance element, element of interaction with the one body, the physical body of the One God, here specifically is a process — of greater relaxation, of sorts.

A person is more relaxed when he is asleep, and it is some kind of a special state, the state of the initial creation of the body. Because initially, when there was just an embryo, in terms of mechanics his state was very simple. When the person was just at the beginning of his creation, for example one day after the fertilization of the ovum — he is basically in a passive state, and therefore the act of the initial conception, which is the state in which he was initially transferred — it is a calm action, that is, some kind of calmness, and therefore he is asleep, that is, he is lying down.

And if we consider cases in which someone can sleep for 4 hours, for example, and then work — and there are confirmed examples of that in history — here it means that the person simply compensates to a greater extent, that he simply interacts more with the physical body of the One God, specifically at the level of cognition. That is, because beyond the elements of cognition he sees His body. At least he knows where the physical body of the One God is located; perhaps not consciously, [not] so clearly, but maybe as a light of penetration, a light of interaction. It does not work in the state of wakefulness, he sort of misses it. And in order for that to happen one has to have a very dense rate of events; that is, people like that, as a rule, do a great deal. With the exception of cases when it is a deviation, but what I mean is that when a person in actual fact does a lot, then as a general rule people like that work a great deal and do not sleep much.

So, why a lot? Because God — He shows through in actions, that is, one body of God as an element of the event. If we understand the organization of the physical body of the One God, we understand, generally speaking, the organization of events. So it would seem: what is so unusual — knowing the physical body of the One God? Since it is by analogy, it should be the same: take the human anatomy atlas and look: there seem to be no problems, so it's clear. But here we are talking about the true original organization, as I mentioned in the case of a truck with a trailer; what is behind the trailer, what is behind the manifested material World? And so when I am now talking about what happens if we are talking about the elements of physical reality — any ones, then the primary element, which, as an acceptor, perceives information or realizes its information — this is blood, which does not flow out, because this is the harmonious setup of the World, and not because the capillaries are trapping it.

In case if we have, for example, the element of absolute protection, say, from bullets, from some external event. Why during wartime in different situations were there people who passed through a hail of bullets without getting as much as a scratch? And that is because the World was set up ins such a way for them that it did not contain elements of external penetration. For example, superconcentration on reaching the goal; precise knowledge of meeting with the One God, in accordance with the agreement. There is precise knowledge there, that nothing will happen — no problems — he just calmly walked along his line, and that's all. So, the line of entrance for the One God (they talk about parallel spaces, world, etc.); so, the line of entrance, in actual fact, according to the logi, specifically in line with this method, is close to the physical body of the One God. This is, in essence, what is already embedded in the person himself — these are his specific actions. Because God is manifested both by actions, and some events. Everything is God.

If we proceed from this point it means, that from this monolith level [follows] the principle of the complete freedom of the individual. The principle is that you have the possibility first to discuss — that is, it may be done, or it may be not done; or you can do it independently, but then you have to crate more. So there is the element of the absolute freedom of the individual; this is constant creation, constructive creation of the subsequent reality. That is, in this case this is originally stated by the One God, and therefore you have no boundaries at all. Therefore, the absolute freedom of the individual lies in infinite creative construction of some subsequent elements of reality.

And from this it follows, that if we consider, for example, the norm of events in the plane of thinking — we shall now proceed to thinking, — then engaging in the processes of control through the elements of thinking, for example, it is possible to enter the system of infinite thinking. Just by saying: this area is an infinite source of energy, information, and so we take it and connect to the task, and it can turn over by itself for an infinite period of time, and it will result, naturally, in attaining the goal. So why it is possible to reach the goal by thinking? Because thinking, in actual fact, — is the sign of subsequent infinite creative freedom.

Why is it always possible by using the technology of control with the Spirit

— consciousness for example — to restore the physical body and to prevent something catastrophe, some catastrophic or similar event; is it possible to prevent even the thought of such an event, negative for you, on the other hand? Because you can, using thinking, transition to the next phase of development. And from here it follows, that thinking — is the next phase of the natural, that is, free development for you.

For example, if you think about the question: from the standpoint of the One God, generally, what is the thinking for? People would resolve tasks at the level of feelings, for example, and in general would be using other mechanisms, for example, using spiritual vision. And everything can be seen, so the person would keep going, he would know where he is going: clairvoyance would make sure there were no problems, for example. Even though clairvoyance as an element of thinking can be perceived from the standpoint of already knowing the laws of the World. Therefore, specifically the thinking, so called reproductive thinking, which creates subsequent reality, is generally the strongest sort of self-purifying mechanism, the mechanism for creating the subsequent reality, and, generally speaking, it is an element of complete freedom, which is a necessary element. That is, we came to understand that even such a familiar phenomenon as thinking is actually a necessary mechanism.

So, when we start getting more deeply into ourselves, and look at this thread of understanding inside, we can see that thinking grows sort of from the inside, it is created within the person by all the organs, all the elements of reality, the whole World; in fact, most importantly — by the Soul, originally. And this is manifested sort of on the outside, that is, as if some behavior program for the specific person, that is, he thought something through and started walking. It is wrong to say that this is a program that was imposed on him: he first thought something through and then started walking. If he is not thinking about the process of thinking and walking, for example, he perceives the situation quickly and does not think through the piloting in some actions, or this is the level, comparable to the level of direct vision, when it is visible without that, and so he walks because it is visible.

But thought is a type of form which is effective, if you think it through. „I am thinking there about this and that“ — and he designates this as a thought. And so it happens that this is simply what we can say, that a person is thinking at all times, but here he may perceive it differently: either as an intuition, but of instantaneous type; or as a form, which is called „thought“, for example they say „an intelligently stated thought“, or something like that. Such statements tell you that the thought may be separated, seemingly, from the spiritual action. But in essence in front of the One God we always have that which for Him is both thought and Spirit, and generally speaking even the Soul consciousness of the person — these are for Him equal systems, besides the fact that He initially singles out the Soul at the level of the depth of his Soul.

Thus, the physical body of the One God has an attribute comparable to us .That attribute is that in general we are mutually recognizable: the Souls of people and the Soul of the One God. And therefore, when we logically single out thinking or Spirit, that is, we separate one fragment from another simply by the logical method, the One God does it by giving us this capability to identify. He also gives us the capability to arrange. So then, what kind of capability is it? What do we use to identify if with respect to other categories, or informational events, we are sort of occupying the external position? Or is the situation here, that if we, for example, have some kind of predefined control, then it is not always informational events only; that there can be initially given events, Spirit, Soul. So this external element is the physical body of the person, that is, God provided the physical body specifically in order to have the external system of analysis and control. That is, this is after all a controlling organ, controlling system, therefore, naturally the One God must have a physical body

— and a human one at that.

And so it happens then (by the way, I brought you to this simply logically, and taking into account that the text of the workshop is created at the moment the words are pronounced, that is, I do not prepare — I simply see what is necessary for the salvation of all, how you perceive that, how others will be saved by this text, these actions — because it is not only text there, but also direct actions of control take place from my side), and therefore we have an interconnected system, that the physical body of the person proves the existence of the physical body of the One God. And when we come to that, the act of faith appears complete; then, naturally, everyone believes and everyone saves, particularly since, for example, there is proof: the resurrection of Jesus, complete regeneration, other systems related to complete regeneration or instances of resurrection.

So it goes that here, if we bring up this topic, we then see the development of infinity, the way it is for real. That is, we can then comprehend that there are stars, and how they are generally organized. That is, we can know any remote Worlds and realities from the standpoint of correlating specifically the movement of approaching the physical body of the One God, at the same time understanding it and its interconnection with external reality. The understanding there is more fine in nature, as I mentioned using the same sauna as an example — it is one that does not have broom with cut branches, the nature is not damaged, etc. And when we start moving towards him, knowing that he is located within the physical body, we just make the task considerably simpler.

From the standpoint of the methodology of control, it looks simply like an arrangement of those peculiar — they look like lines of power — in the direction of His physical body — so that's where the act of faith appears — where the physical body of the One God is located.. That is, to see Him means already to believe. There, naturally, there is no concept of any analysis, because, if you see a person — you believe that the person exists. But it is impossible not to believe here. And on this the true faith is based, the true movement and, generally speaking, true salvation. In terms of salvation, in a broader understanding, it always exists; the question is different: what is the speed of attaining true salvation? One can sail on a ship and seal, for example, one crack or hole, but still — is everything sealed? What is the truth of salvation? And the truth is — when everything is running fine on this ship.

So the concept of the truth of the salvation — is when in fact there are no real problems, and the person will survive for sure, events are definitely coming to a normal situation, and he with certainty reaches the objective of creative, constructive control. Attains that for everyone, including himself, and in the process everyone is saved. Here is the element of both salvation for all and eternal life, another aspect of it is that only by approaching you understand the physical body of the One God. You, at the same time proving that this is an effective mechanism and, as something already self-evident, that he has a physical body and it shows you development, and showing how the physical body of the One God gives you development, you, in fact, create a normal stable World. That is, the physical body of the One God shows in what way you must create physical reality and, generally, how to restore yourself and how to teach others, let's put it that way, etc. Therefore as a control mechanism I suggest that you use this method multiple times on something completely different: elements of reality, including your health, salvation of others, macro-salvation, some target systems for control over physical or informational elements of reality, etc.

This completes my lecture for today.

Thank you for your attention.

GRIGORI GRABOVOI

Selected Lectures

Edition: 2011-1, 27.07.2011

Jelezky publishing, Hamburg 2011

ISBN: 978-3-943110-11-1

NOTES

CPSIA information can be obtained
at www.ICGtesting.com
Printed in the USA
LVOW13s1232060717
540419LV00034B/1140/P

9 783943 110111